Intuitive Eating

A Revolutionary Program To Stop Dieting, Binging, Emotional Eating, Overeating And Feel Finally Free To Live The Life You Want

© **Copyright 2019 - All rights reserved.**

The content contained within this book may not be reproduced, duplicated or transmitted without direct written permission from the author or the publisher.

Under no circumstances will any blame or legal responsibility be held against the publisher, or author, for any damages, reparation, or monetary loss due to the information contained within this book,either directly or indirectly.

Legal Notice:

This book is copyright protected. It is only for personal use. You cannot amend, distribute, sell, use, quote or paraphrase any part, or the content within this book, without the consent of the author or publisher.

Disclaimer Notice:

Please note the information contained within this document is for educational and entertainment purposes only. All effort has been executed to present accurate, up to date, reliable, complete information. No warranties of any kind are declared or implied. Readers acknowledge that the author is not engaging in the rendering of legal, financial, medical or professional advice. The content within this book has been derived from various sources. Please consult a licensed professional before attempting any techniques outlined in this book.

By reading this document, the reader agrees that under no circumstances is the author responsible for any losses, direct or indirect, that are incurred as a result of the use of information contained within this document, including, but not limited to,errors, omissions, or inaccuracies.

INTRODUCTION 6

CHAPTER 1: THE ACT OF EATING 10
Why Do We Eat the Foods We Eat? 10
Why Do We Eat the Way We Do? 17
What Kind of Eater Are You? 19

CHAPTER 2: INTUITIVE EATING – THE PROGRAM TO QUIT ALL DIETS 26
What Is Intuitive Eating? 26
The Psychology of Eating Intuitively 32
Why We Fear Listening to Our Gut-Brain? 35
How to Eat Intuitively: A Step-by-Step Guide to Prepare Yourself 39
How Is It Different from Mindful Eating? 45

CHAPTER 3: THE PRINCIPLES OF INTUITIVE EATING 48
1. Reject the Diet Mentality 49
2. Honor Your Hunger 52
3. Make Peace with Food 54
4. Challenge the Food Police 57
5. Feel Your Fullness 60
6. Discover the Satisfaction Factor 63
7. Honor Your Feelings 68
8. Respect Your Body 70
9. Exercise: Feel the Difference 73
10. Honor Your Health with Gentle Nutrition 75

CHAPTER 4: INTUITIVE EATING STRUGGLES 79
7 Myths and Misconceptions About Intuitive Eating 80
7 Mistakes You Are Making with Intuitive Eating 86

CHAPTER 5: INTUITIVE EATING AND COMMON EATING DISORDERS 92

Anorexia Nervosa 93
Bulimia Nervosa 96
Avoidant Restrictive Food Intake Disorder (ARFID) 98
Binge Eating 100
Emotional Eating 105
Nighttime Eating Syndrome 107
How to Eat Intuitively with Dietary Restrictions? 110

CHAPTER 6: BECOMING AN INTUITIVE EATER 115

The Thought Process of an Intuitive Eater and Dieter ... 117
Raising Intuitive Eaters 120
The Holiday Survival Guide When Eating Intuitively 128

CHAPTER 7: INTUITIVE EATING AND WEIGHT LOSS 135

How Listening to Your Body Can Help You Lose Weight? 136

CHAPTER 8: INTUITIVE EATING FAQS 143

Is IE a Diet? 144
Am I doing it right? 145
Does it Work? 146
What if I also want to lose weight? Is it ideal for me then?
.... 146
I fear that I will only eat junk if I start eating intuitively.
How will I be able to stop? 148
Do I have to be driven? 149
How will I know when I am hungry and when I am full? Is
there some particular way to judge my fullness? 150
How long before I become an intuitive eater? 151
If I am only eating junk what about my nutrition? 152
I have decided to eat intuitively but where do I begin? 153

CHAPTER 9: THE BENEFITS OF IE 155

One Step Towards a Healthier You! 155

CHAPTER 10: IS IT FOR ME? 165

WHO BENEFITS THE MOST FROM INTUITIVE EATING? 165
CONCLUSION 168
FREE BONUS 170
REFERENCES 172

Introduction

What is the first thing that crossed your mind when you first picked up this book? Did you think, "Oh well, another diet that doesn't work," or "Will the food industry ever stop conning us?", or "Well, I might as well try this."

Whatever reasoning your mind came up with, we are sad to disclose that you are wrong! This book is nothing of the sorts.

If you are one of the 45 million Americans who have weight loss as their New Year Resolution then let us tell you, this isn't a weight loss book. Wait, don't just stop reading this, give us a chance to explain what it is if it is not a diet or weight loss book.

So, why did you pick up this book in the first place and how can it help you?

Chances are you picked it up because you haven't lost hope; hope in yourself and your relationship with food. If we were to do a psychic reading just now, we think you picked up this book because you are fed up with all your former diets and just wish there was something that can lead you to a normal and happy life where you didn't have to count every calorie in your food. Or maybe because you have spent the last 10 years of losing and gaining weight but failed to maintain it. Perhaps, you have just had a meal and you're still craving more. Maybe you picked up this book because you are obsessed with a certain food group say, desserts or beverages and you can't seem to stop. Or maybe you want to get out of binge and emotional eating patterns.

Whatever your reasons may be, let's get one thing clear, shall we?

This book isn't only about weight loss, it is also about eating healthy and nutritious food. It isn't about yo-yo dieting but rather a complete guide to embrace healthy eating behaviors. The purpose is to give you a break from dieting and help you start living your life like you should be. The goal is to allow you to see past a diet and experience what it feels like to have a diet-free life for once.

In this book, together we will go on a journey of a lifetime where not only will we tell you about intuitive eating but walk you through each step you need to take to become one. Talk about being a good partner!

With intuitive eating, you will learn how you can listen to your body's inner cues of hunger and fullness. With intuitive eating, you will realize that food can also be a source of pure joy and pleasure. With intuitive eating, you will reconnect with your body and honor it with the right nutrition. You will learn how to manage your cravings and recover from eating disorders.

You will learn about why you haven't been able to eat properly for as long as you can remember. You will learn that no matter how hard you try, chances are 95% of the diets will fail you. Don't believe us? Let us prove it to you right now!

You will also learn that diet culture is anything, but a myth and you certainly don't have to look a certain way to gain your partner's attention or a new suitor. Hell, ditch him if, even if it's one time, he tells you that you need to change who you are!

Once you are done doing that, come back to read more about how this is going to be a revolutionary change, maybe not as big as the Apollo 11 to Mars, but no less for someone with a bad relationship with food.

So, are you all set for the biggest change of your life?

Yes!

Say it louder, we can't hear you.

Yes!!

Louder than that...

Yes!!!

Wow let's begin then!

Chapter 1: The Act of Eating

In this first chapter, we are going to be talking about the science of food, how we choose amongst different foods, what factors differentiate between the food we like and don't like, why we eat the way we do — sometimes in three meals and sometimes six — why we keep failing at diets or more precisely, why do they keep failing us, what kind of eater you are.

Interesting, no? Well, how about we make it more interesting with some amazing research work over the years to determine the likelihood of you picking an apple instead of an orange. You may not realize this but there is a ton going on behind this decision of yours and we are going to break it down for you below.

Why Do We Eat the Foods We Eat?

It isn't as simple as we eat because we are hungry. In his book tilted *Mindless Eating: Why We Eat More Than We Think*, Dr. Brian Wansink, a renowned food psychologist studied the consumption patterns of humans and why they eat the way they do. According to Wansink, we unintentionally make about 200 food decisions every single day! However, we aren't even aware of 90% of them. We are going to be looking at some more thought-provoking studies found in his book to help us understand better.

Cravings for Bad Food

One of the key features of nearly every diet ever created involves complete abstinence from some food. Sometimes, it is bad carbs, proteins or even dairy! This is where the fault lies. Human psychologists suggest that the more we are told to abstain from something the more we crave it. So, now you know why it is so hard to put that big slice of cake back in the fridge. This behavior is even prevalent in kids. How many times did you tell little Jimmy to not put his finger in the socket? Does he stop? Yeah, we know!

So basically, every time someone tells you that you need to stay away from something when you are trying to shed a few pounds, they are setting you up for cravings for that exact same thing.

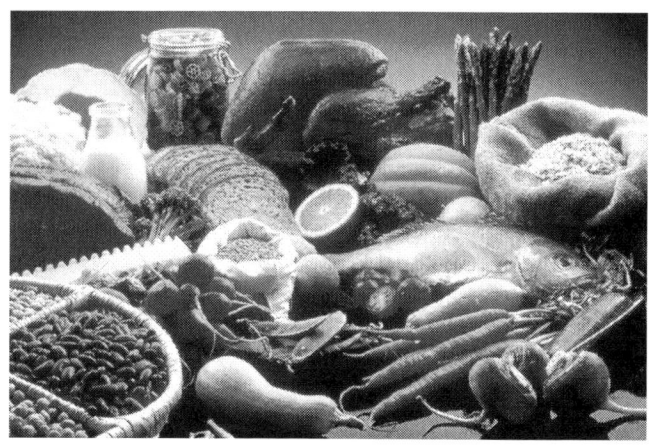

Cheap Vs. Expensive

According to another study that put all the wine experts to shame is the difference between the expensive and cheap wine conducted by a Ph.D. student named Frederic Brochet at the University of Bordeaux (Morrot, Brochet, & Dubourdieu, 2001).

In the experiment, Frederic argued that the branding of what we buy has a lot to do with the perception we have of it in our minds. In his study, he gathered 57 participants and served them with a red Bordeaux from a midrange bottle with a label that referred to it as a modest vin de table.

The same participants were called back a week later to try another bottle of red Bordeaux from a high-end bottle with a label that termed it as grand cru. The participants were then asked to rate their experience of the first wine and the second. A majority of them rated the first wine as weak, unbalanced, and simple. The second wine from a different label was rated as complex and balanced. The most shocking thing was that the wine in both bottles had been similar. Frederic called this perspective the expectation that most of us have towards certain brands. Although they are serving the exact same thing, we tend to believe that they are somehow better than the competition since they are expensive and look more sophisticated.

Here's another crazy study in which the researchers asked some participants to try out a cup of flavored yogurt but in a dark room. The researchers had specifically told the participants that the yogurt was chocolate flavored even though it wasn't. It was strawberry flavored.

Surprisingly, 59% of the participants rated the chocolate-flavored yogurt as having a mild and subtle strawberry flavor that they loved the most. So you see, just because they were told something all along, their minds tricked them into thinking it was.

This is what the marketing industry is built upon. Breeding that very perception in our minds that despite knowledge, we tend to overlook the obvious and give in. This is also how most of your favorite celebrities are earning viewers when marketing diets, makeup or beauty treatments. They assure you that you need them to look better and more like them, which isn't true.

Presentation Matters the Most!

Be it in Master Chef or your favorite restaurant, a lot of times it comes down to how well a dish has been presented even if it is as simple as mashed potatoes or a slice of cake. The art of presentation does have a positive impact on our brains and boost hunger.

This very phenomenon was studied in this next research where the experimenters presented brownies in three different ways (Grabinsky, et al., 2015). However, everyone was getting the same brownies to taste. It was just the presentation that differed. Participants were divided into three different groups.

- The first group was presented brownies in a china dish.
- The second group was presented brownies on a paper plate.
- The third group was presented brownies on a tissue paper.

The experimenters then asked the participants how much they will be willing to pay for the brownies.

- The first group said that they would pay $1.27 for each piece of brownie.
- The second group said that they would pay 76 cents for each piece of brownie.
- The third group said that they would pay 53 cents for each piece of brownie.

This means that the presentation does have an appeal on our brain and purchasing. No wonder we always go for the shiniest thing in the store just because it seems more tempting to have.

Who Wants a Hershey's Kiss?

In an experiment, Wansink conducted on the secretaries in an office. He found that when they sat near a clear dish of Hershey's kisses in comparison to an opaque dish filled with the same, they ate more. Furthermore, they gained five extra pounds over the year. It was calculated that secretaries sitting near a clear dish of Hershey's kisses consumed 77 calories a day (Wansink, 2005).

The point, in case, was that whenever something is placed in front of us, we tend to incline towards it, even when we aren't hungry. The presence of it tricks the mind into thinking that it is craving for it. And it happens with everyone. Whether it is a boxful of donuts in a police station or a bag of chips in your lounge, if you see it, you are likely to eat it.

Up for Some Popcorn, Anyone?

Another interesting experiment in the book also reveals that when we are given a large portion of something, we eat more. Yes, we are talking about that hearty steak meal you get at your favorite diner with a side of mashed potatoes and veggies. In a study, Wansink gave some moviegoers the choice to opt for a medium or a large size of popcorn tub. Despite saying that the size didn't matter, moviegoers with the larger tub of popcorn ate 53% more than those with a smaller tub. This proved that when we are presented with something in large quantities, we eat more of it, even if we aren't able to finish it all.

Why Do We Eat the Way We Do?

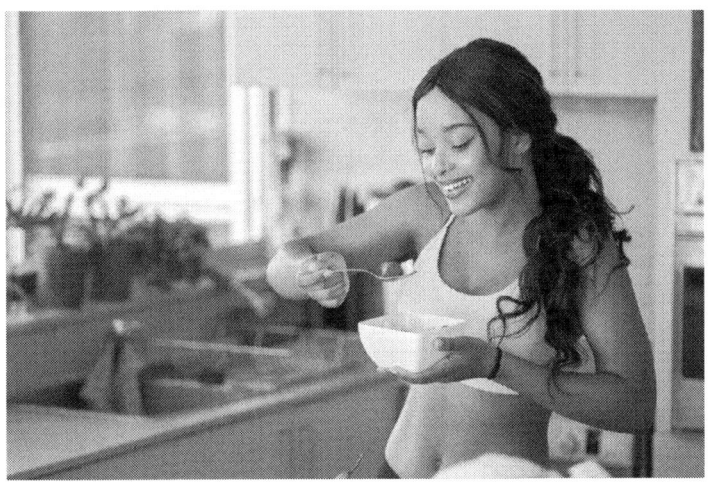

Coming to the second important aspect of why we eat the way we do, many researchers believe that our age, gender, lifestyle, family history, and hormones have a lot to do with that. Published in the *Journal of American College of Nutrition*, the IFIC Foundation research aimed to identify the factors that impacted on the way we eat so that we can understand how we can make changes and adapt to better and healthier lifestyles.

The research discussed what exactly we wish to achieve when we eat the things we do and whether it changes with our age, gender or body mass index (BMI).

Approximately 2,700 American adults participated in an online survey from age 18-80. The survey was demographically charted and consisted of 6,689 drinking and eating occasions the participants reported during the day before.

Astonishing results surfaced which defied the previous assumptions about how we eat, how often we consume food and drinks, and why we preferred them over the others. It was believed that the decision to eat had to do with the lifestyle characteristics of the participants. Age was another important factor that helped the researchers understand why we eat the way we do. Seniors were more likely to plan their meals as per schedule than adults and teenagers. It showed that they used the time of the day as a trigger rather than hunger itself. If they had lunch at 12:00 am every day, they resorted to that time only.

Secondly, it was also believed that moderation in eating and drinking also contributed to why we eat the way we do. The respondents stopped eating when they felt satisfied, had enough, or when their plate was empty. However, this moderation differed for every individual.

If we take this research as a beacon of guidance, we realize that the reason we eat isn't entirely based on hunger but rather motivated by factors like the presence of food, time or habit. This can help those trying to manage their weight as they can focus on the factors that trigger eating and thus avoid them.

What Kind of Eater Are You?

Now, here's the next important thing. What kind of eater are you determines what practices you adopt when it comes to eating. Do you confide by time or are you walking with a spoon in your pocket all the time? Do you prefer a proper setting or any place is good for you as long as you get something to eat? Are there any restaurants you prefer for hygiene basis or do you base your food choices solely on taste? All these questions will help you understand your eating habits and whether they need to change or not.

Confused? Keep reading and you will understand what we are talking about.

Emotional Eater

Are you someone who, every time watches The Notebook cries with a pint of Ben and Jerry's in your bed? Are you someone who eats just because they are bored and have nothing else to do? Do you treat yourself with a drink every time you finish a report before its due date out of sheer happiness?

If all these sound like things you do, you are an emotional eater. You are someone who eats according to their mood and not their hunger. You celebrate with a bottle of whiskey and dig your spoon into ice-cream when you're sad. All your eating habits revolve around how you feel. There isn't much care for rational thinking before you pick something up. This often leads to eating more when you see your weight creeping and being unable to fit into your skinny jeans. The cycle goes on and on until you move to hazardous and stringent diets that do you more harm than good. An emotional eater just eats to satisfy themselves.

Critical Eater

A critical eater is someone who either has set preferences on what they eat or nothing at all. They are an all-or-nothing kind of individual. Critical eaters are obsessed with diets despite knowing the nutritional importance. They usually have a hard time sticking to just one diet as they expect fast changes. When they don't happen as per their set goals, they give up and move onto the next one. They have this preset notion that dieting makes them a conscious and good human being which means that when they are not on one, they consider themselves as bad. They give in to the temptations of delicacies but regret it later by going on strict and restrictive diets that sometimes has consequences.

Habitual Eater

As the name suggests, a habitual eater is someone who indulges in bad food choices, giving themselves the excuse that they will only try it once. They know the importance of eating right, maintenance of an eating routine and preferences, but sometimes, they are derailed by responsibilities and time constraints. One of the biggest disadvantages of being a habitual eater is that habitual eaters don't eat when they feel their appetite building, instead, they eat because they are used to it. They might say something like, "I will have dinner by 7:00 p.m. and not a minute late. After dinner, I will not eat anything till the next morning." This mentality of eating at a fixed time prevents them from listening to their internal cues.

Energy Eater

Imagine someone with a granola bar in their hands as their breakfast and they can't shut up about the benefits it holds. Yes, we all have that one colleague in our office or a friend in our social circle. Energy eaters are all about quick fixes. You will always find them talking about the nutritional facts of things and their favorite, on-the-go snacks throughout the day. The only problem, however, is that they eat too much of them. Although there isn't any harm in eating energy fixing food, an excess of it can be counterintuitive. A majority of energy bars and foods come packed with calories that our bodies may not require. In fact, sometimes, instead of trying to eat healthily and consume fewer fatty foods to avoid calories, we eat more of them found in granola bars. Besides, they also increase insulin production in the body, which isn't good for your overall health and leads to making you feel hungrier.

External Eater

External eaters wait for external cues to eat. Oh, it's a colleague's birthday? Bring in the cake. Oh, it's a baby shower, let's get your hands full with the sugary delights placed so elegantly on a platter. Such external cues trigger their hunger and not their body. Their brain awaits for such signals to occur so it can trigger hunger. These people are the worst to hang out with as they will stop at every cupcake shop or roadside hot dog stall because they are tempted to eat. This can result in overeating without the eater even realizing and later suffering from digestive issues and complaining about it to you.

Sensual Eater

A sensual or mindful eater appreciates whatever is presented in front of them. They don't just eat the food, they devour all the flavors and spices in it sensually. They will moan at how juicy that steak is, they will give a shout out to the waiter for the delicious wine, and later leave a thank you note for the chef who made the red velvet cake. The point here is that they love to explore the food involving all their senses. They are in no rush to finish up and chug everything down, instead; they relish in the exploration and deliciousness of it. Unlike critical or picky eaters, they don't always think about making rational decisions when it comes to food.

Chaotic Eater

A chaotic eater is someone who will eat whatever they can whenever they can. They skip meals frequently and usually eat on the run. They also have little memory of what they ate or when which means they either starve their bodies or overeat. They don't plan or schedule their meals and don't have any specific preferences either. This usually results in them gaining or losing weight overtime — both of which impact their overall well-being and health over time.

Restrictive Eater

A restrictive eater is also similar to a critical eater as they are very particular about the food they eat. They are mostly on diets and have journals listing their calorie intake for every meal. They also follow a strict choice of food and have a list of items they can and can't eat. They don't give in to the temptation of what lies in front of them. If you know of someone who is a restrictive eater, you may have spotted them weighing their meals, reading labels of products and charting them. Since they are so strict about their food options, they often fear eating food prepared by others or with others. Even before they are finished with their current meal, they start worrying about their next one.

Intuitive Eater

Intuitive eaters are different from any of the eaters mentioned above. They wait for physical cues from their bodies. They don't indulge in mindless eating and only eat when their body tells them too. They rarely give in to temptations. They also look for cues to stop eating to prevent overeating. They experience no guilt and have trust in themselves when they are around food. But this doesn't mean they don't enjoy their food because they do as there are no restrictions about what to eat or how much to eat.

Take Away

In this chapter, we take a look at our connection with food, what motivates or stops us when it comes to choosing between different food groups. Later, we also discuss why we eat the way we do and how sticking to a fixed schedule to eating is doing us more harm than good and why the practice must be made obsolete. Finally, we tried to categorize people into different categories of eating from restrictive eater to an intuitive eater.

Chapter 2: Intuitive Eating – The Program to Quit All Diets

Researchers at the University of California published a report in the 2017's edition of the *Journal of American Psychologist* which aimed to understand and monitor the long-term effects of dieting. The study proposed that 66.6% of dieters didn't lose weight over five years dieting all the way and in some cases even gained more weight. Whenever we come across such statistics, they reinforce the idea that conventional diets may offer desirable results for the short-term, but they aren't the way of life. The restriction to certain foods and the addition of others only causes a misbalance. This is where intuitive eating comes in.

What Is Intuitive Eating?

A term or phenomenon coined by two Californian nutritionists Evelyn Tribole and Elyse Resch; the intuitive eating program is listening to your body's innate need for food. It involves biological wisdom that each of us possesses but fail to pay heed to. According to the originators, our body already knows what food and nutrients it requires. It also knows when to eat, when to stop, and the best habits to adopt concerning food. It is a better judge by miles in comparison to the dietary recommendations that the majority of the diets and its practitioners rub in our faces.

Intuitive eating program steers away from rigid dietary requirements and scientific explanations and lays value to the psychological need for eating. When we begin to eat intelligently, we try to find that lost inner wisdom and let it guide us to ensure that our body remains healthy and well-fed.

What led to the discovery of the idea were conventional dietary programs. The developers of the idea questioned why diets failed to work. It was thought-provoking that despite the many conventional diets available in the markets, Americans weren't losing weight. The obesity rate in the country continued to rise. Furthermore, the developers also discovered that dieting had a major consequence which they termed the diet backlash. The diet backlash refers to an observation that dieting for many years led to multiple eating disorders and promoted guilty, compulsive, binging, and self-loathing behaviors in many. This was because whilst diets promoted the usage of certain foods, it also asked the dieters to restrict from some. The restrictive foods were of course more delectable and crave-able, which only led to frustration upon rejecting it and guilt upon giving in to its temptation.

To further prove the point that intuitive eating was true, the only suitable way, the originators cited a 1991 study by Dr. Leann Birch. It was published in the *New England Journal of Medicine* and revolved around the eating habits of children. According to the research's findings, children have the innate ability to regulate their habits around eating. They can also do so in a healthy manner. This meant that parental control over what they should eat and what they shouldn't was in fact, counterproductive. Some other studies also confirm that the additional pressure from parents to eat right has led to bulimia, anorexia and other eating disorders in teenagers and children. This is a common sight to behold in participants taking part in beauty pageants from an early age. They are made to follow a strict diet and denied all pleasures of what being a kid comes with. In some studies, it has also led to issues with self-esteem and self-loathing. Coming back to the original study, if the children do possess that innate wisdom to eating right, there must be some way to rekindle it within them as they grow older and allow it to blossom so that healthy choices can be made.

Lastly, the originators of the intuitive eating program also registered that no matter how well-conceived a diet is, it only has short-term implications. This isn't the case with intuitive eating. In fact, intuitive eating shuns all such beliefs that dieting is good for you and encourage you to listen to your body's needs and accept the way you look. It also promotes the health movement and strongly believes that health conditions like poor dietary habits and obesity leads to increased risk of diseases and illnesses.

So, if we were to summarize the hyped concept of eating intuitively, we have the following four domains.

Relying on Satiety Cues

The first crucial area in an intuitive eating program is to establish trust in your innate hunger and wait for the satiety cues. Let these cues guide your eating behavior. How does it differ from conventional dietary restraints? It differs in the way we let our internal cues determine our eating regimes instead of our external cues. For instance, the majority of diets propose that one must break down meals into five to six smaller meals per day. However, there is no such limitation in eating intuitively. You must eat when you feel hungry and how much you should eat must depend on your calorie-burning capacity and metabolic rate.

Quitting to Eat for Emotional Reasons

Secondly, in intuitive eating, you look for the physical reasons for eating rather than solely relying on your mood or emotions. Intuitive eating implies that one must only eat when their body shows physical signs of hunger such as a growling stomach and also stop when it feels full. This disregards two very important notions with diets, for example, overeating and eating because you are overwhelmed with emotions.

You Don't Need Permission to Eat

Unlike most fad diets that clock your meals, there is no such concept in intuitive eating. This domain involves your willingness to eat whenever hungry and refusing to label foods as good or bad. When you eat as per your own body's schedule and needs, you prevent overindulgence and the shame and guilt accompanying it.

Not Categorizing your Food

In this last but important domain regarding intuitive eating, you begin to realize that every food has a purpose to serve. Be it any vegetable, fruit or protein, each has its own benefits for our bodies and must be taken without restrictions. However, the context of the situation may vary.

The Psychology of Eating Intuitively

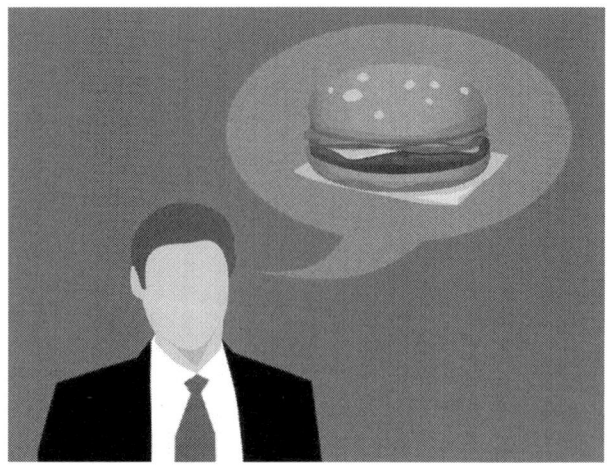

Imagine waking up in a world where your relationship with food was easy. You ate the things you love, at whatever time you felt hungry, stopped eating when you're full and leading an active and healthy life. Alas, in the real world, it isn't this easy. So, who has made it difficult?

You!

Yes, it is you who has made the eating process so calculative, restrictive, and scheduled. Imagine if you continued to eat the way you are supposed to, there wouldn't have been any moments of guilt or being hard on yourself. There wouldn't have been any beating yourself up later when your stomach got upset or you put on weight. There wouldn't have been any eating linked to how you felt — happy, sad, angry or stressed.

Think about just eating for the sake of eating and providing your body with the nutrients and energy it requires. Is it that hard?

Not really.

Believe it or not, but the picture we presented at the start of this section can be your reality if you want it to be. Your relationship with food should be based on trust. You should be able to trust your body to signal your cues when to eat and trusting it to tell you when to stop. Once you begin to make well-informed decisions regarding your food, you won't have to rely on fad diets anymore.

But how does it actually work and what is the psychology behind it?

Intuitive eating is a scientifically proven phenomenon. It works, in the same manner our inner gut works. Have you ever had déjà vu or feeling like something wasn't right? Perhaps, you are walking down a dark alley and feel like someone is stalking you? Or felt your heart beating faster when you are with a loved one or meet your favorite celebrity for the first time? Ever had that uncomfortable pinching in your stomach when you didn't feel sure about something? Have you ever gotten all sweaty and shaking when you're going for a job interview?

What is it if it's not your body's enteric nervous system signaling you? Science refers to it as our gut-brain. Odd, but we do have a brain in our belly too. This gut-brain differs from the brain we have in our heads but works in the same manner, more or less. The enteric nervous system lies in between the muscle layers of the esophagus, small intestine, and the stomach just under the mucosal lining. There is a complex network of neurochemicals and neurons that help teleport any messages and signals our gut-brain is suggesting.

Researchers believe that our enteric nervous system is constantly throwing out suggestions and giving information about your nutritional needs to the brain. However, since we are so used to listening to the external cues, we often miss hearing it. Think about it, how many of us eat when the lunch hour begins? Or when our parents call us down because the dinner is served? Or when we are hanging out with friends or a partner to dine out? The first rule of eating intuitively is listening to the internal messages and honoring and trusting them to make decisions regarding your food.

Why We Fear Listening to Our Gut-Brain?

If listening to your gut-brain is as easy as paying attention to a speaker in a seminar, why can't we all do it? There are a few fears involved.

For starters, most of us believe that by listening to our inner cues to tell us what we should eat and how much, we might resort to unhealthy eating behaviors and end up making the wrong choices. Who knows if we are decoding the signals the right way? What if we end up overeating and gaining weight over time? This sounds sensible but it is also bad judgment. This arises from the lack of trust we have in our body and the natural cues it is capable to give us. But you can't be blamed for it entirely either. We have been brought up this way and it is hard to give up after so many years, isn't it ladies? Of course, regaining trust with your relationship with food involves just you, and it can seem hard. If only there were some counselors to guide us through the process and rekindle that lost spark. Okay, maybe we went a little off-road here.

Coming back to our original point, it will take time to rebuild trust in your body and take an ounce of patience on your part. But it is worth it in the end. If you stick to it forever, you will never have to go back to dieting again.

The worst thing about any diet is that it promotes the elimination of some foods. However, did you ever realize that the foods you aren't allowed to eat are also the ones you crave the most? And what's even worse is that you didn't even want them before you started the diet. For instance, let's say you don't have a sweet tooth. You come across a diet that restricts any sugar content. You think to yourself, "Great, I don't even like sweets that much. This would be so much easier to pick." A week down the lane and you see this stunning layered chocolate lava cake in the hands of a waiter serving it to a couple next to your table in a restaurant and you feel something within you. What's that? A craving? But you didn't feel this way when you saw a chocolate cake before. Then why all of a sudden you want to fork it down your tummy? Somehow you still resist the temptation and tell yourself that once you are done with the diet, this will be the first thing you will have. And you do! In fact, you overindulge in it, having it more often than before. And then in no time, you see the dropped pounds creeping back up and you are right back to where you started.

It is very natural for your body to crave the things it has been restricted from. The longer you put it off, the more intense your cravings will become.

With intuitive eating, there is no restriction which means no cravings. Every food is allowed and thus, feels normal. When you reach this point where you stop experiencing sudden cravings, you are on the path to becoming an intuitive eater. It is important to understand that cravings don't always happen for fast food, carbs, and sugary delights. It can even happen for the simplest of foods. Picture this, you are traveling to a different country on vacation. You are excited to try the local cuisine. You do and for some time you find it tantalizing as well. But after some days or perhaps weeks, you will miss the cuisine from your country. You will be surprised that you will be craving for food you called boring and sad and hated when it was made it your home. So basically, we just don't crave the things we can't have but also the things we do, and it all comes down to having a variety of everything. This is what intuitive eating programs preach.

They tell you to listen to your body's hunger cues and what it is craving. When everything is consumed in a natural and limited manner, your body will resort to a weight that feels normal. This is referred to as the body's set-point weight. Let us help you understand it with a very basic example. Imagine you placed water in a container and kept it out. When you first kept it, it was at room temperature. If the weather outside in the daytime is sunny and warm, the water's temperature will increase after a few hours. During the night, the weather changes and it becomes chilly. The water's temperature will decrease. Hunger and metabolism operate in the same manner.

Hunger cues and metabolism plays a crucial role in our body's regulation of weight. We only feel hunger when our weight falls beyond our set-point weight. Metabolism also slows down in case energy is required. However, when we feed ourselves and feel full, our set-point weight goes up and the rate of metabolism increases to bring the body back to its set-point weight.

How to Eat Intuitively: A Step-by-Step Guide to Prepare Yourself

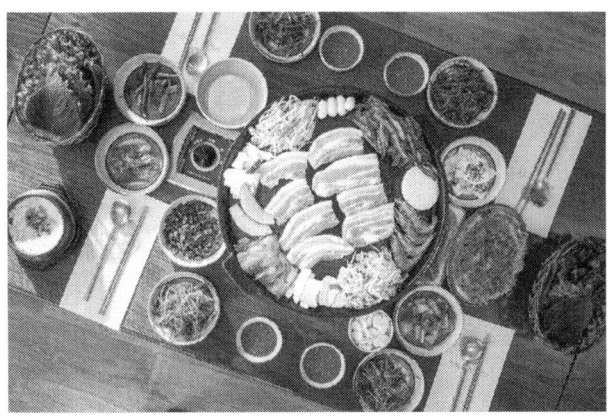

Now that we have covered the majority of what intuitive eating is all about, it is time we actually learn how to implement it in our lives to start listening to our body's natural responses and maintaining a healthy weight without having to give up on something. We have broken it down into six simple steps to get you into the intuitive eating mode and prepare yourself for a better change in your lifestyle.

1. Have Realistic Expectations and Accept the Way You Look

First things first, we are all beautiful in the eyes of our loved ones. People who really love us, love us for who we are including the way we look. Besides, we were born to stand out and thanks to our unique genetic blueprint, we do! Then why do we always want to join the crowd and become invisible? Doesn't sound too ideal, does it, ladies?

So, if you have a few extra pounds hanging around your waist or have a double chin, that doesn't necessarily mean you aren't healthy, or you need to change the way you look. Of course, change is a requisite when your chubbiness gets in the way of your health and increases your risk of certain diseases. If not, then there is no reason to keep trying to reach an unsustainable, unrealistic and unhealthy weight.

You need to set realistic goals and expectations when starting with intuitive eating. Since it isn't like most diets, you are less likely to observe the results overnight. Setting the bar too high for yourself will only sadden you later when you fail to hit the mark. Besides, a good eating habit shouldn't involve stress and harm to your self-worth. You need to be accepting of the way you look and stop beating yourself about it. The sooner you let go of the guilt that makes you want to try on different diets every now and then, the better off you will be — physically and emotionally.

2. Understand That Fad Diets Aren't Going to Work

If your main concern is to lose weight, it may seem tempting to pick a diet that promises guaranteed and quick results. However, this weight loss is usually temporary and comes with many drastic measures such as radically cutting down calories, eliminating food groups or sticking to low-carb diets only. Since these measures are quite challenging and directly attacking the body's natural biology, they lead to cravings in the long run. Moreover, there is always a chance of falling off the wagon and feeling guilty and self-doubt.

So, the more rational thing to do here is to rely on a food routine that has worked for people for centuries and includes eating real food in moderation and moving around. When preparing to eat intuitively, you must look for nutrient-enriched diets that promise steady energy levels, a stable mind, and a healthy body. You must choose foods that honor your health. You must eat things that satisfy your hunger and taste buds and make you feel good and energetic.

3. Shun the Good or Bad Thinking About Food

Some foods are more nutrient-dense than others but that doesn't mean you should eliminate them completely from your diet. Doing so will only add to your stress levels of not having that forbidden food and increase your craving for it. If you are trying to become an intuitive eater, you need to make peace with food, stop fighting, and settle for a truce. Now, this doesn't mean that you go all out on processed goods because that is what you crave. You still need to prioritize foods that are healthy. However, you can always have them in limited quantities if the craving doesn't go away.

If you keep telling yourself that you need to abstain from certain food groups completely, it will also lead to feelings of shame and guilt in case you end up breaking your vows. Researchers believe that a mentality of all or nothing gives rise to binge eating. Those who give in to the temptation of their craving often end up having more of it and later regret their decision.

Your goal shouldn't be to strive for perfection here, but rather progress. Consistently eating healthy should be the ultimate goal without having to give up on your favorite comfort foods. Moreover, you need to stop labeling food groups as good or bad or black or white. You need to establish a balance between the two and aim to have more of the healthier foods than the unhealthy ones. This way you won't have to feel guilty about having your favorite foods or eating them in large quantities.

4. Eat When You're Hungry, Stop When You're Full

We have already discussed this several times above that intuitive eating promotes eating when your body asks for it and then stopping when it is full. There isn't any room for overeating or eating out of habit if you are trying to become an intuitive eater. This will also help you honor the food in front of you as you feel blessed to have it and discourage overeating or overindulgence. When you make this a habit, you will begin to notice that you will no longer crave food and only eat when your body tells you to.

5. Don't Use Food to Handle Your Emotions and Stress

Yes, we understand, there is hardly anything more satisfying than downing a whole cheesecake while watching Bridget Jones Diary because you feel like that is you. Just because of a bad date, breakup or anxiety due to a tough and unappreciated work life, you can't always go to food for comfort.

Emotional eating may seem like the best choice, but it is only going to make your situation worse. How so? Because then you would also have to deal with the guilt and shame that creeps up after you are done with your comfort food and have a stomachache. If you are wondering what should be the alternative, then you already know where this is going. Eat intuitively!

For a majority of people, eating intuitively opens doors to new possibilities to deal with stress without resorting to fatty, oily or carbs-dense foods. If you are looking for means to cope up with your stress and emotions in a healthy manner, start an intuitive eating journal or download intuitive eating apps that are readily available in the market today. Jotting down the amount of food you eat, how you felt after its consumption, and how many calories it has can all take off some stress and guilt that usually builds up when you don't eat intuitively.

6. Fill Yourself with Sufficient Calories

Got a bridal shower to attend or is it a high school reunion? We get it, you want to look your best and those few extra pounds you put on over the holidays are just adding to your anxiety. Of course, you want to lose them but resorting to temporary quick-fixes and fad diets aren't the solution.

Experts believe that when we suddenly deprive our bodies of say, calories, it lowers our energy levels and slows down our metabolism. And the pounds you shed will come back in less time it took you to lose it because it will be mostly water weight. So, it may seem like it will work short-term but with consequences that can and will be long-term. Depriving your body in such a way will make you fatigued, stressed out, and feeling discontent.

How Is It Different from Mindful Eating?

A lot of people who are new to intuitive eating think of mindful eating and intuitive eating as the same. Although they can't be used synonymously, there are several similarities between the two. Some researchers go as far as suggesting that neither can exist without the other. Then why the different names and different approaches?

In this section, we are going to be looking at the many similarities and differences between the two and then let you decide if these two works in unison or not.

Starting with the similarities:

- Both mindful eating and intuitive eating are approaches to eating without the concept of dieting. They both strongly believe that the diet culture must be eliminated, and healthy eating should be promoted.
- Secondly, they both encourage forming a healthy relationship with food and not simply eat for the sake of eating but rather enjoying and seeking pleasure from it.
- Thirdly, they both have been used as a tool for weight loss and proven effective in the long-term.
- And lastly, there is no judgment when it comes to what you are eating or how much you are eating. The goal of both these approaches is simply to promote the consumption of the healthiest, nutrient-dense foods to lead a healthy lifestyle.

Although there aren't any major ones, the subtle differences between the two include:

- Where mindful eating opens your curiosity and encourages you to notice and appreciate the food in front of you, intuitive eating is more concerned with your body's needs.
- Where mindful eating can sometimes be used as a tool to measure and limit how

much you eat, there is no such restriction with intuitive eating. Intuitive eating allows you to eat to your heart's content and be a little mindless about it.
- Where mindful eating preaches open-mindedness, intuitive eating is more about rejecting the diet mentality and culture.

Take Away

In this chapter, we covered the basics of what intuitive eating is all about, why we should adopt intuitive eating, the science behind it and a step by step guide for beginners planning to get started. Next, we addressed a common misconception about intuitively eating where many people thought it was synonymous with mindful eating. Therefore, we compiled a list of all the similarities and differences to help the readers distinguish between the changes and understand intuitive eating more aptly.

Chapter 3: The Principles of Intuitive Eating

Have you ever wondered why we adapt to the diet culture? What made us rely so much on them that we are willing to sacrifice our basic body's needs for it? It all started when our parents strictly told us to finish everything on our plates. Leaving even a pea behind was never an option whether we were hungry or not. We were told to drink milk and abstain from sweets. In fact, some parents didn't even allow their kids to devour the candy they collected on Halloween. We were then told that some foods were good for us as they helped us grow and some were bad and must be avoided. When all that happened, we stopped listening to the internal cues from our bodies and listened to the external ones instead. Society is to blame as it taught us how much we should eat, what we should eat, and what to avoid. Had it not been this coercing, we might have had a completely different looking body and health.

The ten principles of intuitive eating discard this notion and list down ways we can have a healthy relationship with our food and body. Let's take a look at what they are and how we can incorporate them into our lives to live a fulfilling and diet-free life.

1. Reject the Diet Mentality

Did you know that 95% of diets fail? But if we are going to be talking about the failure of diets, it is crucial to understand that it isn't the diet that fails, but the people who fail at diets. There is a vast difference between the two. Research has shown that dieting for a long period can have drastic consequences on our health and well-being. Since most diets expect their followers to go against their biological needs, it often leads to you questioning about your internal intuition. Moreover, every new diet somehow affects our level of confidence as well and is accompanied by guilt when we fail to keep going. This sets in feelings of unworthiness where you feel like you are an outcast and a disgrace to your own self and society.

Thus, when you reject the diet mentality, you free yourself from all the fatigue, shaming, obsession, yo-yo, and failure. And the best part, it isn't very hard to adopt either.

How to Reject the Diet Mentality?

Here's how you can reject the diet mentality and move towards a diet-free and guilt-free eating lifestyle.

- **Identify what really is the diet mentality**

It often feels like the entire fitness and wellness industry is making money off your insecurities and imperfections, doesn't it? They target the weaker ones and urge them to spend hundreds if not thousands of dollars into fixing themselves. In today's world, obsession and idolization regarding your health have become a norm. You don't even realize that you are surrounded by it completely and falling into its trap one step at a time. It is high time that you see it for what it is and recognize that you don't need to be a part of it. You are better off without it and not going to lose your hard earned money to the big corporations.

- **Distance yourself from things that promote diet mentality**

Since the goal is to eliminate this culture the first thing that you need to do is distance yourself from all those things that encourage dieting in the first place. This involves unfollowing all those diet accounts, people, and celebrities on social media like Facebook or Instagram who post their everyday routine workout sessions and diet plans and talk about all those expensive products, supplements, and training they used to look the way they do!

Secondly, unsubscribe to all those email reminders that pop up suggesting a sale on a weightless supplement and how you can save money by buying a year's worth supply. You don't need that.

Thirdly, unfriend all those people who constantly put you down over the way you look. Nobody has the right to tell you what you should do, eat or what you should wear. Your body is your temple and only you get to decide what it needs.

- **Learn about the long-term dangers of dieting**

We have linked several studies in the previous chapters that suggest that dieting does more harm than good. Take note of those studies and educate yourself. Let your mind make a rational decision about what is good and what isn't.

Dieting is one of the many reasons that lead to binge eating. Ever been to a party where you just can't put your spoon down and keep asking for seconds? If so, that is what dieting does to you. You overeat and purge on food.

2. Honor Your Hunger

The second principle demands that you honor your hunger. What does that actually mean?

Honoring your hunger means that you wait for the cues your body will most likely signal when it's time to eat. By honoring your food, you teach your body to eat not only foods that are available but also foods that it is asking for. For instance, if you feel like indulging in a big cheesy burger, don't try to shrug off the need with something else. Instead, have that burger and let your body know that you will continue to nourish and honor its needs as long as they are sensible and healthy. This involves building a trusting relationship with your food and body.

How to Honor Your Hunger?

- **Educate Yourself About What Hunger Feels Like**

There are several ways hunger is felt by someone. Sometimes, it is that growling feeling you get in your stomach which feels as if someone is twisting it. Other times, it is that lightheadedness that suggests that you are running low on energy. Then there is abdominal pain, irritability, fatigue, inability to concentrate, weakness or preoccupation with food. All these are cues that our body uses to remind us that we need to eat.

However, if you still aren't sure that you are getting mixed signals from your body, track your time with food. It takes about an average of 4-6 hours for your body to digest food. This means that you should feel hungry after 4-6 hours. But this isn't set in stone as our bodies are different from one another. Also, it depends on what you have consumed in your last meal as some foods take longer to digest.

- **Calculate Your Hunger and Fullness Scale**

Since we all feel and express hunger in different ways, it is only fair that we all have our personalized hunger and fullness scales. A hunger and fullness scale is a scale with two extremes. Think of it as a 1 to 10 scale where 1 represents most hungry and 10 most full. You need to rank your hunger and fullness based on these figures. If you are at one, you are starving to death and if you are at 10, you can't take another bite of your food.

Ideally, your hunger and fullness scale should range from 4 to 7. This way, you are eating before you are too starved and finishing before being physically full. Remaining in the in between will eliminate the physical discomforts such as lightheadedness or bloating and gas when you're too full.

Feed Your Body What It Is Asking For

When you feed your body the sustenance it wants, you are building body trust. However, if you still wish to remain on the healthier side of the spectrum, the best way is to keep foods that are healthy in your pantry and fridge. Another way to do so is to prep your meals in advance so your body already knows what it's going to get in a few hours and will most likely crave that.

The ultimate goal should be to honor your hunger. This means that if your body is craving cake, don't try to substitute it with a cookie just because you think it would be unhealthy. That is cheating and not honoring your hunger.

3. Make Peace with Food

This next principle allows you to consume all the food groups in your repertoire without penalizing yourself with guilt and shame. It also means you have complete authority to eat as much as you want as long as you don't overstuff yourself and eat things that are medically restricted. If you live by this principle, you are going to detach labels from food. They will no longer be good or bad. You also need to realize that no food is going to make you a bad person, unhealthy, addicted or rampant. By doing so, you are letting go of any need for binging or eating emotionally. You understand that all foods are available and up for grabs whenever your body feels. When you try to make peace with your food, you don't just eat everything in one sitting. You see it as a journey of giving up on food rules you have engraved in your mind and unlearning and exploring new foods, what they taste like, and their importance. Here's how you do this.

How to Make Peace with Food?

The first thing you need to do is begin with making a list of all the items you don't like. You can even rate them from somewhat likable to least likable. Once you have a list, pick one item from it and buy it for the sake of trying it. Purchase it in multiple servings so that you are just not eating them because intuitive eating tells you to.

This is a practice that inculcate the message in you that no food is good, bad or off-limits. All foods serve a purpose, including the one you dislike. Be it a pint of ice cream, a bag of chips or broccoli, they all have calories that your body requires to gain energy. Maintaining a balance between the things you like and things you don't will keep your nutritional levels in place and you won't have to make any sacrifices by ditching the things you occasionally eat that are delicious or never eat because they are disgusting!

Next, time your meals. You need to be mindful of whatever you are eating in a place free of distraction. You also don't need to be extra slow or fast like you are in some sort of a rush.

And finally, sit down to finish the meal using all your senses. You may want to journalize all the feelings you have while you eat whether it is pride, guilt or shame.

4. Challenge the Food Police

What is a food policy and how can you challenge it? The food police are all those thoughts that determine what foods you should eat and what foods are bad for you. Sadly, the media has shaped our minds into making that distinction, preventing our internal cues to decide what is best for us. What follows is shame and guilt when we have something from the forbidden food group when it shouldn't be. This food policy is always critiquing us on our choices and making decisions for us. The food police can take the shape of your parents telling you to slim down or no guy will ever find you attractive or a friend who doesn't want you to look fat at her wedding because you are the maid-of-honor. But most of the time, it is our own thoughts that become our biggest enemies and dictate our choices for us.

When we quiet the food police and listen to our internal bias, we allow ourselves a rare opportunity to make good decisions based on things that are pleasurable and satisfying. This is what this principle is all about! Do you want to learn of ways you can challenge the food police? Look below.

How to Challenge the Food Police?

- **Don't make judgments**

Although we have been repeating the mantra of eating whatever you want and whenever you want, this doesn't mean that you have the full liberty to ignore all nutritional values and indulge in foods such as processed meats and fizzy drinks. It is true that you have the freedom to choose, but you are also expected to act mindfully.

So, you start with observation without judgment. Suppose you are consuming protein without any fruits or veggies. You don't need to think constantly that this is bad or judge your food choice. You also don't need to think about how much you will need to run on the treadmill just so you can burn off the calories. You also don't need to make up for the meal you had by having ONLY fruits and veggies at dinner.

What you are doing is judging instead of enjoying and savoring your food. Even if it is an oily steak, it still holds important nutritional value. Even if you are at a dinner party or wedding that has a hearty and calorie-rich menu, you don't need to feel guilty about eating it or not. This principle teaches us that you need to stop judging your food choices, especially when it is your body that is craving for the meal. And you certainly don't need to punish yourself for it later.

- **Don't aim for perfection the first time**

It isn't a movie where the first time you try eating intuitively, you become the best at it. You need to keep practicing over and over again until you get it. Intuitive eating takes time and patience. Since you can't stop eating, don't think of it as a one-time gig that you can gloat about with your friends on your next brunch. Instead, think of it as a lifestyle change and its implications on your life. Besides, you have your whole life to figure out your body's needs. This isn't a race, and no one is chasing after you. So, instead of diving right into it and expecting to come out victorious and a perfectionist, see it as a gradual process with positive results.

If the food police are getting on your nerves just because you had too many donuts last night at your promotion party, remember that not every day will not be like that and it is okay to take out some time to have fun with food. You don't need to beat yourself up because of that and then stay away from donuts for a whole week. A day's eating isn't going to make you fat and it certainly shouldn't demotivate you.

- **Get support from friends to join your team**

Since changing your eating habits will be difficult at the start, how about you get some of your friends to fight off the food police? Since there aren't any hard and fast rules to follow when eating intuitively, having a support group will only make it more fun and less of a regime. Share the ridiculous rules that most diets want you to abide by and talk about the things and actions that lead to self-pity, emotional eating, shame, and guilt concerning food choices.

5. Feel Your Fullness

This step involves complete awareness while you're eating. Once you decide to eat intuitively, you need to get rid of your previous habits around food. For instance, if you just came off a diet or meal plan that you had been practicing for months, you may find it difficult to identify when you are full. Therefore, before we talk about this in detail, understand that it is going to be a process and you will keep learning as you go along. Feeling your fullness isn't about demonizing fullness, but to chart how you feel after the consumption of various foods, and you can keep in mind this question: Are you able to differentiate between the different textures and tastes without judging yourself?. Feeling fullness is also a blessing in disguise as you remind yourself about the availability of food which prevents overeating. This is especially important when coming off a restrictive diet as your chances to go on a binge is at its highest. It is also pivotal to note that it is okay to eat when you are extremely hungry, even if you just had a meal a couple of hours ago. However, you must remember to stop eating before you feel full. This is how you respect your body's cues by not quieting its demands but also not going all in. This balance between the two extremes is what this principle is all about.

Below are some great ways to get you started!

How to Respect Your Fullness?

Before you begin eating, chart how hungry you are. This will help you time your next meal and also allow you to keep track of your fullness when you feel it.

As important it is for you to be physically hungry, it doesn't mean you need to starve yourself before your next meal. If you wait until you are too hungry, you will not be able to track your fullness when you reach it as your mind will still be too tempted by the food that is in front of it. The likelihood of you overeating will increase and it isn't something you want.

The next important thing that you should note is to avoid eating when you are distracted. When you are planning to start eating, ensure that you have switched off your TV, placed aside your phone, and you're not distracted mentally. Did you know that you eat 25% more when you're watching TV? It is also best to minimize the conversations at the dinner table as it will make it harder for you to time and track your fullness.

There shouldn't be any rushing with food. It isn't a race. You don't have to munch everything down before the lunch hour is over. Take your time, slowly biting and savoring each bite. Ideally, you should take out at least 15 to 20 minutes for every meal. Doing so will allow you to take note of your fullness when you reach it and prevent overeating. This is only possible if you listen to your gut-brain carefully and read the cues your body signals.

Use the fullness scale to measure how full you physically feel after a meal. Did you reach complete satisfaction or not? If yes, then by how much?

Next, you need to drop the "clean your plate" mentality. If you feel full when your plate still has food on it, there is no obligation that you must clean it. Listen to your body instead of listening to external pressure. You need to stop when you feel full.

Allow yourself to have some compassion and grace. Since intuitive eating is a gradual process that takes time and practice, forgive yourself if, at some point, you pass comfortable satiety. There will be days when, despite being intuitive eating, you will overeat or feel uncomfortably full. So, don't beat yourself up about it. Intuitive eating is all about forgiving yourself and letting go.

6. Discover the Satisfaction Factor

Discovering your level of satisfaction is all about finding pleasure in eating again. You may be wondering how this principle is any different from the principle #5. Here's how. This principle is about finding the distinction between being full and being satisfied. Has it ever happened to you that despite being super full, you still have cravings for certain foods? Like you want to eat more but your stomach thinks otherwise. If yes, then this is the difference between being full but not satisfied. This also happens when we substitute something for something else. You really wanted to eat a cheeseburger with fries, but you ate a salad instead because your diet tells you to. Do you really think you will be satisfied at all? Yes, you will be full, but not satisfied.

Intuitive eating forbids this. It suggests that you eat the one thing you are craving for instead of those ten other foods you eat because you are bound by some rules. Not only will you feel happier and satisfied, but you will also save yourself from the angst. What you eat shouldn't just be about filling your stomach, it should also fill you with content and joy. The only way you will feel it is if you eat whatever you want. If you need help to better understand whether you are satisfied with what you ate or not, here are a few tips to get you started with.

How to Feel Satisfied After a Meal or Snack?

- **Step 1: Talk to Yourself**

The first step involves asking yourself what you're really craving. Next, sit down and think about this for a minute: what drives most of your food choices? Is it some external pressure or the food police? Then try to recall the last meal where you truly felt like you treated yourself with the best? How long was it? If you can't even recall the last time you had something you really wanted to without following those diet rules, then you don't experience satisfaction often.

Don't make your next meal the same. Think about what you really want to eat right now. Is it grilled cheese, a pizza or a slice of cake? Whatever it is, just remember to stop eating when you're full and aim for a middle spot on your hunger and fullness scale. Satisfaction should be the goal.

- **Step 2: Think About the Food Mindfully**

Once you have sat down for a meal, don't just gobble it up like a robot. Instead, indulge all your senses into it. This will elevate your experience and make you feel better. It's really like foreplay and the anticipation. The more you have it, the better you will feel later.

Think about how it looks, how it smells, and what it tastes like. Is the temperature right? Does its texture excite you? The more explicit and detailed you are about the food, the more satisfied you will be.

- **Step 3: Think of It as an Experience**

Remember, you aren't just eating; you are also enjoying it. How will you be able to enjoy it? When there are zero distractions in your way. Limit the casual chit chat whilst eating: find an ergonomic chair to sit down and eat, get all your required cutlery in front of your beforehand, have a glass of water beside you, and set aside any gadget that might distract you with a pop-up message. The goal is to allow yourself to tune in with your body and go on an exciting journey together. Savor every bite and notice all those feelings that arise within you every time you take another bite. You must also cut down any judgments that keep humming into your ears that what you are eating is going to make you fat.

- **Step 4: Check-in with Yourself**

Lastly, do check in with yourself. An ideal time to eat and enjoy food is when you are mildly hungry. When you are starving to death, your first instinct is to chomp down as fast as you can. If you aren't hungry at all and eating for the sake of eating only, you won't be able to enjoy it. If, at any point you realize that the food you are eating doesn't excite you anymore, stop. This is what the originators of the intuitive program call the last bite threshold. When you reach the last bite threshold, even the most exciting of foods become your "normal" and you no longer enjoy it. Therefore, stopping at that point is a must. Besides, you can always have more of it when the craving arises again.

7. Honor Your Feelings

Although eating for emotional reasons is looked down upon in most diets, there is something remarkable about it too. When you eat to cope with stress or emotions, at least you acknowledge that there is something wrong and needs attention. Instead of eating, you can sit down and think about those feelings and try to resolve those problems that trigger emotional eating in the first place. Moreover, you can even look at other ways to cope with your feelings as the emotional eating is often accompanied by shame and guilt later. So, if you want to save yourself from all that, consider this a heads up. The next time you feel sad, stressed or just down for no reason, don't think of food as your savior. It may make you feel better for some time, but it does have some unlikeable consequences. So, leave that bottle of wine for a happier occasion because if you don't, you are going to wake up with a massive hangover that will make you hate yourself even more than the previous night.

How to Cope Without Food?

If you are looking for some other ways to cope with your feelings, here are some great tips to get you by.

- **Seek Nurturing**

Tribole and Resch suggest that to cope with your emotions, it is best to seek nurture from something other than food. When you are occupied with other means of nurturing, the thought of eating loses its appeal as your needs are met. Think of food as a part of the healing process but not the default answer for everything. All you need is some encouragement and nourishment which can easily come from:

1. Taking a nap to forget about the problem
2. Listening to some relaxing tunes to distract your mind
3. Taking a long shower to treat yourself
4. Meditation to really think about the problems, their root cause, and possible solutions
5. Getting a spa facial, massage, or manicure

   and pedicure

- **Acknowledge Your Troubles**

You need to acknowledge the things that are troubling you. Will they go away without bringing food into it? Sometimes it is okay to not feel okay. You can always pick up the phone and dial a friend's number and ask them to come over. Or you can confront the issue or the person that is making you feel that way. You mustn't always think of food as your go-to medication.

- **Distract Yourself**

If you still don't feel better after a consultation or confrontation, try moving away from it by tricking your mind into doing something else. If you think that you might not be able to resist eating, the best way is to remove yourself from the place where you have easy access to it. For example, if you are at home feeling low and you know there is food in the kitchen. What do you? Go for a walk or on a drive. Or pick up a book or get cleaning. Distractions not only take your mind off your troubles; they often serve as a means to reduce the intensity of it. An hour ago, you might have felt like crying your eyes out, but now after Marie Kondo-ing your room, you might not feel that way. The feelings of sadness will still be there but less intense. The less intense your feelings, the less likely you are to go near food for comfort.

8. Respect Your Body

Although body love is equally important to practice, this principle is more about the liberation of the body rather than self-love. This is about you accepting the way you look, your height and weight and features. It is about acknowledging the fact that we were all made different and regardless of trying hard to look like someone else, say your sibling, your neighbor or a model on the cover of Vogue, we need to seek acceptance about the way we look. Of course, there isn't any harm trying to look better, but not at the stake of your mental and physical health. Therefore, wishing that you were a different height or shape means you don't respect your body the way that it is. This principle is also about ditching the fatphobia culture in society and aims to see everyone as they are without the weight stigmas. If you don't respect the body you have and continuously feel like some diet, supplement or physical activity is going to change it, then it will be difficult for you to practice intuitive eating as you will be constantly worrying about weight loss and your overall appearance.

How to Respect Your Body?

- **Keep It Hydrated**

Drinking more water should be your primary goal. A hydrated body is full of energy. The skin feels better, the organs function smoothly, and it makes you feel less hungry all the time. This is one of the most important ways to honor your body to prevent any digestive and kidney-related conditions.

- **Get Enough Sleep**

Standardly, your body needs at least 5 to 7 hours of sleep every night. A lot of times, we compromise our sleep for things like workout, work, and household chores. However, a lack of sleep has its side effects as well and they take no time to show in a fatigued, sluggish and cranky you. Besides, what's the point of a workout if you aren't allowing your body enough rest to recharge itself for another day? Thus, the second most important way to honor your body is to get a good night's sleep. If you suffer from a sleep disorder, do try taking short naps in the afternoon to cover up for the sleep lost at night. A good night's sleep does wonders for your body, mind, and skin, so try to honor your body with it.

- **Appreciate Your Body**

Next, you mustn't forget to appreciate what your body does for you from carrying your weight to functioning properly to make you feel like "you" every day. Think about it, if it wasn't fit or weak, would you have been able to accomplish all that you can?

- **Limit the "Fat" Talk**

Limit the negative talk about the way you look. We all talk bad about our bodies. Some of us want to have a bigger chest, while others want their thighs to look thinner. No good has ever come from talking about your flaws unless you are willing to make a change for it. Besides, even with all those flaws, your body doesn't let you down, so why do you?

- **Go Shopping**

Since it is all about honoring your body, how can we not mention clothes? Honoring your body also includes dressing it in the right, well-fitted clothes. We have to find a balance between too fitted or too loose. Basically, wear what looks good and compliments your body without making it compromise. Dress comfortably, so that you allow some room for your body to breathe freely.

9. Exercise: Feel the Difference

There is no compulsion for you to hit the gym every day when adopting an intuitive approach. However, a sedentary lifestyle isn't encouraged either. Keep your body moving so that it doesn't develop a sluggish or hunched posture with time.

If you do opt for some physical exercises, opt for the ones that are sustainable and enjoyable. Don't waste your time trying to do exercises solely for burning fat or losing weight. instead, pick something you enjoy or else you won't be able to do it for long.

How to Become an Intuitive Exerciser?

To get you started, here are a few tips:

1. Respect the needs of your body and listen to the internal cues and triggers. For instance, if running on the treadmill causes chest pains, don't continue with it. Chest pain is a clear indication that your body isn't ready for running.
2. Think of fatigue as a cue as well. If some strenuous high-intensity interval training (HIIT) is leaving you with zero energy levels throughout the day, then maybe you need to tone it down and try something less intensive and hardcore to build your stamina first.
3. Next, you need to have a purpose for exercising. Why are you doing it? Is it to lose weight, burn calories or simply stay active and healthy? The more convincing your reason, the likelier you are to continue with it.

4. Expand your options when it comes to exercises. Don't just go for a jog or work on your upper body area only, aim for a variety of exercises so you continue to enjoy the mix and don't think of it as a workout. For instance, if you are into sports like tennis, boxing or cricket, these can be exercises as they keep you on your toes and include movement. So, if you aren't the gym-type, try taking up a sport you enjoy and consider it as your physical activity.

10. Honor Your Health with Gentle Nutrition

Although, the very approach of intuitive eating encourages us to eat whatever we feel like, it doesn't mean that you can put everything in your body. Oxymoron, right? Well, the researchers Tibole and Resch wanted the practitioners of intuitive eating lifestyle to suggest that whenever we feel like eating anything, they must evaluate the nutritional value of it. Good nutrition must still be one's top priority. You must make food choices that are healthy in general and honor your health. Thus, think about incorporating more fruits and vegetables or try having them as a side dish to some protein or carb-dense food. Trying this approach won't make you completely get rid of food that you really wish to enjoy, but it also has some nutritional value to balance out the unhealthy fats.

How to Honor Your Food with Gentle Nutrition?

What does honoring your food with gentle nutrition actually mean and how do you do it? Think of this as an amalgamation of all the principles we previously covered.

This last principle is all about expanding your options by giving your body the choice to choose from a variety of foods with good nutritional values. Indulge in foods that make you feel good without any judgments but are also good for your body. It is also about becoming more aware of your body's needs. Honoring your food also means that you listen to your body's reaction to all the foods you eat. Learn how it reacts. When your stomach hurts that means that the food you consumed didn't sit well with your body, thus, you might want to hold back on that particular food. Similarly, if after the consumption of a certain food, and you feel not only do you feel happy but also more energized and focused, then you might make this food a staple to your meal.

Next, you need to find a balance between not eating enough and not eating too much.

Keep in mind that there are no forbidden foods anymore. You can have all that your body craves without feeling guilty or trying to substitute it for something much healthier. Every food has some nutritional value, so don't try to always aim for those that rank highest on the nutrition chart and be full but not satisfied.

And lastly, don't be too hard on yourself. There will be days and events where you eat more than you should have, but that doesn't mean that you need to go on a diet for the rest of the week to balance out the extra calories. It is okay to have some less than stellar days. No one is judging you except yourself. Sometimes, it is okay to not be a rude critic and let go.

Take Away

This chapter takes a detailed look at each of the 10 principles of intuitive eating that serves as the basis of the overall approach to eating. From honoring your hunger, fullness, and body, it also covers aspects like the importance of good nutrition, the role of physical activity, how one can get started with intuitive eating, coping with emotions other than with food, and how to quiet the food police and so much more. This chapter not only describes each principle in its core essence but also teaches how they can be implemented in daily life, so you can reap the best results.

Chapter 4: Intuitive Eating Struggles

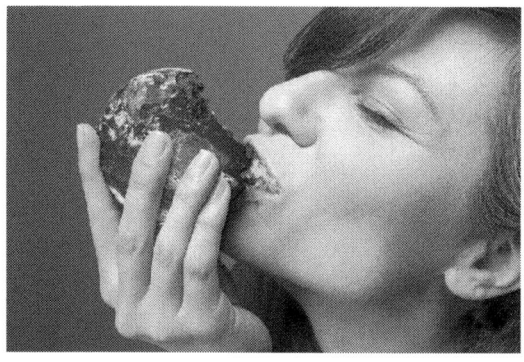

A dieter may say that a diet is a solution to all your problems, but an intuitive eater will tell you that all the answers you seek are within yourself. It is true, all the answers we seek are within us because it was designed by Mother nature that way.

Call it a Buddha approach, but this is exactly what intuitive eating teaches us. The idea behind intuitive eating is to reconnect with our inner self, tune into it to let us guide ourselves with its wisdom and help us figure out a way to eat the right way.

Unlike traditional diets, intuitive eating allows its followers some wiggle room to interpret their body needs and execute them. This is what makes it such an ideal approach to eating. There are no limitations or bindings. However, it is the same flexibility that makes it so easy to give up on intuitive eating as most people consider it a failure as it doesn't make them lose weight. But it was never the actual goal of eating intuitively. Many people see it as unrealistic because there aren't any restrictions, which they consider a requisite to any diet form.

In this chapter, we are going to be looking at some of the most concerning myths, and mistakes that people make when it comes to intuitive eating and hopefully change the views of those who regard it as a failure or unrealistic.

7 Myths and Misconceptions About Intuitive Eating

Myth #1: Eating Like Children = Eating Junk Food

Just because intuitive eating permits that we pay heed to our cravings, it doesn't necessarily mean that we will only crave junk food. The premise of eating intuitively is to go back to how you were supposed to eat, just like a child does. People often mistake it for only junk food. Ask yourself ladies, has your child ever showed interest in some vegetable or fruit? Do they always want a French fry or sweets? Yes, they may want more of them but not always.

When intuitive eating tells you to eat like kids, it mostly means to eat only when you are hungry and stop when you are full — just like kids do!

Myth #2: There Is No Structure with Intuitive Eating

Again, this is just a myth. Intuitive eating has the most flexible structure if you are interested to know as it allows each follower to tailor the principles as they see fit and as per their individual needs. There is no one way to eat or drink, there isn't a set time when you should eat, and there aren't any restrictions either.

True, there aren't any hard and fast rules like nearly all diets have, but isn't that what makes it unique and adaptable? If someone needs some guidance, they have the 10 principles to get started. Once you work your way around them and follow them passionately, then there comes a time when you no longer need to abide by any rules and regulations and eat whenever you want.

It can be slightly challenging to adopt at first, especially for someone who has a history of yo-yo dieting, but it's not impossible.

Myth #3: It's Much Easier Than Dieting

Wrong, it is much harder to adopt. Why? Because unlike most diets that come with a given set of rules and regulations that the follower must abide by throughout the designated period, intuitive eating comes with no such pamphlet of instructions. It is challenging because it rejects the diet mentality — something we are so used to for ages. There isn't any prize associated with it either. It involves changing your old food habits and adopting new ones. It is about changing your attitude towards food which is difficult. Laid out rules are much easier to follow through as they promise some benefit or prize in the end.

Myth #4: It Is for People with an Eating Disorder

It is for everyone wishing to eat healthier, beat cravings, and set themselves free from the shackles of fad diets. It especially works wonders for those coming off of an eating disorder as they usually have a difficult relationship with food. Intuitive eating is all about mending that relationship and help the survivors get back on their feet and eat healthily.

Many people also think that intuitive eating isn't for people with eating disorders. Although, it is true that when people suffer from some health condition or disorder, their hunger and fullness scale isn't accurate or perceivable. There are days where they may feel hungry all day and then days where they can go for 12+ hours without food.

Even then, it doesn't mean that intuitive eating isn't ideal for them. Intuitive eating is more than just living by the hunger and fullness scale. There are many other principles of intuitive eating that can be adopted such as exercising, making peace with food, honoring the body, respecting its needs, and not giving in to the temptations of emotional eating.

Myth #5: Intuitive Eating Isn't for You If You Have Dietary Restrictions

Thinking that you won't be able to adopt the intuitive eating approach if you have dietary restrictions is another common myth amongst newbies. In fact, it is also one of the most commonly asked FAQ on many online forums and discussions. If someone suffers from a dietary restriction, say lactose intolerance, then they must ensure that their eating intuitively doesn't come in the way of the restrictions. Yes, they will have to honor their body by giving up things with lactose, but it doesn't mean they can't practice all the principles of intuitive eating. They just have been cautious of their cravings and ensure they don't cause any disrespect to their bodies by eating something that is not good for their body.

Myth #6: You Have to Give in to Every Craving That Comes Along

It may seem like it does promote eating whatever you want and whenever you want, but it also promotes eating things that honor your body. How can one honor their bodies? By choosing things that are healthier and more fulfilling with nutritional value. When people begin eating intuitively, they begin to realize that their cravings go away after a while. This happens because they never starved their body when a craving arose and ate whatever it craved. When you stop limiting yourself from something, the urge to have it diminishes as well. It's a lot like when you want that scarf from the jewelry shop that is out of stock. You keep refreshing the website every few days to check if it is back in stock. And then one day when it finally is, you buy it. Then you wear it enthusiastically for a few weeks or months and then it just becomes another staple in your closet that you will soon forget about.

Cravings work in the same way. They hold their charm as long as they are restricted. Intuitive eating is more about deciding what your body needs rather than controlling your food choices. Besides, if you practice intuitive eating or are in the process of becoming one, you honor your body and its needs. At the same time, you also begin to make sound judgments about your food choices. Instead of simply giving in, you understand why you have that desire and where is it coming from. Is an emotional setting driving it or is it more of physiological hunger?

Myth #7: You Are Eating Intuitively Because You Have Given Up

If you think that someone around you has opted for intuitive eating is because nothing else seemed to work, then you are absolutely wrong. Yes, they may have given up, but not on themselves, but on the diet culture that pressurized them to continue with fad and unhealthy diets so they can look like those cover girls. They gave up on the culture that kept telling them that they were somehow flawed and not good enough. If that is the case, then a good thing that they gave up. They are now on the route to physical and emotional happiness.

7 Mistakes You Are Making with Intuitive Eating

Did you know, the number one reason that all these misconceptions and myths form is because we make multiple mistakes with intuitive eating? As long as we don't understand the core concept, we will fail to practice and incorporate it into our daily lives and become an intuitive eater like we were when we were kids. Therefore, to put the above myths to rest, it is pivotal that we take a look at all the mistakes we make while trying to eat intuitively to be able to practice it better.

Mistake #1: Thinking You Can Eat Whatever You Want Whenever You Want

Yes, intuitive eating allows you to pick whichever food your body craves and wishes to eat, but it also reminds us to treat our body with honor and respect. How do you do that? By ensuring that you feed it with good nutrition. Now, if you are following the diet to the tee, you will stop craving junk food as you realize that it leaves you feeling lethargic and sluggish. You want to feel energetic, satisfied, and fulfilled which can only come from healthy eating and limiting the greasy, fatty, and "fast" food along the way.

Mistake #2: Not Giving Up the Diet Mentality

How many times will we have to remind you that intuitive eating isn't a diet? One of the primary reasons people give up on intuitive eating is because they see it as a means to lose weight. Yes, it helps in doing so but it was never its core intention. The core intention was to get in touch with our inner selves and let it take control of our eating choices and habits. If you didn't come with this intention in mind, then perhaps, it is true that it won't work for you.

You need to give up on the diet mentality, which also happens to be the first principle of intuitive eating. The more you cling to it, the lesser your chances of becoming an intuitive eater. You need to trust your body and let it guide you. You need to appreciate the way it looks rather than trying to change it with poor dietary choices that lead to health conditions and hormonal imbalances.

Yes, it may seem difficult to not think about the diet mentality or let it go, but you must if you wish to become an intuitive eater.

Mistake #3: Believing You Can't Lose Weight with Intuitive Eating

There is tons of research, later discussed in chapter 10 of the book, which proposes how remarkable it can be to help you lose weight. If you recently just came off a diet, your biggest worry right now must be if you will continue to lose weight or worse, will you regain all your lost weight. Here's the thing with intuitive eating, if you pay attention to your body's needs and only eat when you're moderately hungry and stop when you're moderately full, you will see the pointer on your weighing scale fall back. Moreover, since there will be no restrictions as to what you can eat, there will rarely be any cravings. If you continue down this road, you will also begin to notice that your body will stop craving for fun foods as it was naturally designed to function on fruits, veggies, nuts, and other nutritious foods.

All these aspects of intuitive eating make for a classic weight-loss recipe, doesn't it? So how can you not lose weight with it?

Mistake #4: Continuing with Food Restrictions

When eating intelligently, there are no restrictions on what you are eating and in what quantity as long as you eat when you're hungry and stop when you're full. There are no rules with intuitive eating which means you can quiet the food police that tell you what to eat and what not to eat. Try to eat more of the foods that pass the health test and are loaded with nutrients like vitamin, iron, Omega-3, and good carbs.

Besides, when you stop denying your body certain foods, it will also put an end to your cravings which often result in binge or emotional eating.

Mistake #5: You Disregard Physical Activity

Just because you are no longer keeping a check of calories with every meal doesn't give you the right to become a couch potato and give up exercising. Staying active is a crucial part of intuitive eating. You need to burn what you are eating and that means sweating up or making your heart race faster for at least 30 minutes per day. It doesn't have to be a hardcore, rigorous fitness regime, but definitely something that gets your blood gushing through your veins faster.

Start with something you enjoy doing, say walking and then pace it up to brisk walking and later full-on jogging to build your stamina and improve your digestion and metabolic rate.

Mistake #6: Thinking It's About Failing or Succeeding

There is no concept of failure or success in intuitive eating. It isn't a race but rather a process that takes time and practice to learn and live by. Despite this, most people just assume that since they aren't losing weight, the diet is a failure and move onto another one. If you keep thinking this way about intuitive eating and stay focused on just the results, you will always be judging and critiquing your choices.

Intuitive eating isn't about perfectionism but rather continuing to progress towards a healthier lifestyle. So don't be too critical of yourself and don't stand on the weighing scale every single day hoping for a miracle. The miracle is learning to listen to your internal messages.

Mistake #7: You Think You Have a Free Hand with Portions

Portion control may not be the core concept of intuitive eating, but there is a strong emphasis on stopping when you're full which is almost the same thing. Since intuitive eating isn't a "diet," many people believe there aren't any restrictions when it comes to portions. True, you can eat whatever you want but in a considerate amount. Though, don't go measuring how many bites you have taken. Listen to the inner cues that tell you when to stop. With time, you will notice how good you become at controlling your portions and stopping when you are no longer hungry.

Take Away

In this chapter, we take a look at the various myths that revolve around intuitive eating and set the score right. Next, we looked at the many mistakes intuitive eaters make when their just starting out. this consists of things like not knowing when to stop, thinking it is only about eating, not honoring your body with the right nutrition, and underestimating the importance of exercise.

Chapter 5: Intuitive Eating and Common Eating Disorders

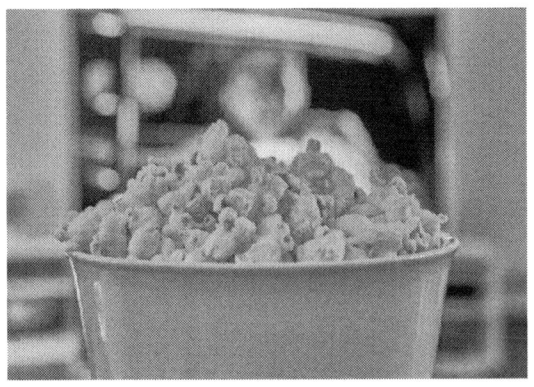

Eating disorders are a combination of illnesses that include irregular eating habits, posing a serious concern about your weight and shape. Disturbances in eating with either excessive or inadequate intake of food are what lead to a disorder. Eating disorders can develop at any age and both men and women are equally at risk. Eating disorders are most common among teenagers and adults, mostly developed due to social media or psychological pressure from society. There are a number of medical, therapeutic, and nutritional treatments to stop and recover from eating disorders, intuitive eating being one of them. In this chapter, not only will we take a look at some of the most common eating disorders but also learn how intuitive eating as a treatment can help recover from them. The reason eating disorders need to be addressed is because they usually coexist with multiple other health conditions like substance abuse, anxiety or depression. Therefore, recovery from an eating disorder is the first step to treating other crucial disorders like depression and substance abuse.

Anorexia Nervosa

This is commonly known as anorexia, and it is an eating disorder that involves an abnormally low body weight. If you know of someone suffering from anorexia or are anorexic yourself, your biggest fear and concern is gaining weight. You have a distorted weight perception and have been eating restrictively for months or years. You indulge in extreme efforts to continue looking for a certain shape and having a certain weight. You have given up on carbs completely, exercise excessively, are misusing diet aids, laxatives, enemas and vomit your food after consumption. Although you already have a significantly low body weight, you still live in the fear of gaining weight and never stop and accept the way you are.

Causes

There isn't just a single explanation of what causes anorexia. It is a complex lifestyle and arises from a multitude of emotional, social, and biological factors. Perhaps, the most prominent cause is our infatuation with thinness today. Ever seen Victoria's Secret models? As much as you adore their figure, it isn't ideal. In France, they have put a ban on models walking the ramp that are too thin as it gives other women unrealistic expectations about how they should look. Some other factors that contribute to developing this eating disorder include:

- Perfectionism
- Low self-esteem
- Body dissatisfaction
- Emotional difficulties
- Strict dieting
- History of physical or emotional abuse
- Troubled past

Symptoms

How do you know if someone is anorexic or in the process of becoming one? There are several signs and symptoms they depict commonly. These include:

- Restrictive eating
- Being underweight or rapidly losing significant weight over a short amount of time
- Obsessing about calories in foods
- Being ritualistic with food such as hiding it, cutting it into short pieces or avoiding to eat in a social gathering
- A continued fixation about recipes, cooking, and food in general
- Depression
- Thinning or loss of hair
- Amenorrhea
- Feeling cold
- Development of tiny hairs on face and body
- Preferring isolation and withdrawal from family and friends

Where Intuitive Eating Comes In?

Since it is a serious condition, medical treatments and therapy have proven most effective as recovery methods. However, since the obsession with food restrictions, calories counting, and weight loss is concerning, an intuitive eating regime can also help in the process of recovery. Since intuitive eating encourages eating when one feels like it, doesn't forbid any foods and promotes a healthy weight and shape by listening to internal cues, it can greatly help the patient recover and restore a healthy body weight by implementing the principles of the intuitive eating program.

Bulimia Nervosa

Bulimia nervosa is another concerning the type of eating disorder in which the individual suffers from a mental illness characterized by repeated binging and purging episodes. In the simplest of terms, think of it as a really bad on and off relationship with food. The individual doesn't know when to stop eating and continues to eat despite being full. Women with bulimia often have a hard time channeling their food-related urges elsewhere and always look to food when they are emotionally or mentally unstable.

Causes

Although the exact cause is still unknown to medical experts, countless research and patient history deduce that one's personality traits, eating patterns, and thinking have a crucial role to play. There are also some environmental or biological factors involved. Like anorexia, it also starts with one's dissatisfaction towards their body. Bulimics are extremely concerned about the way they look, and their body appears. It is also common to notice that those who suffer from bulimia nervosa have poor self-worth and the fear of gaining weight never leaves their minds.

Symptoms

Someone suffering from bulimia nervosa depicts a number of unique signs and symptoms. These include:

- Weight fluctuations
- Damaged blood vessels under the eyes
- Electrolyte imbalances
- Enlarged glands under the jawline and in the neck
- Oral trauma
- Chronic gastric reflux
- Inflammation of the esophagus
- Chronic dehydration
- Infertility

Where Intuitive Eating Comes In?

When recovering from bulimia, patients are encouraged to see intuitive eating as a healthy habit to adopt. It is prescribed so that the individual is able to reestablish a healthy relationship with food, their mind, and body. However, learning to eat intuitively for any bulimic patient is both difficult and stressful. They can't adhere to the 10 principles if they continue to depict the behaviors associated with bulimia. Since the patient had been binge eating for long, it will be difficult to understand hunger cues and prevent eating mindlessly every few hours. They will also need to track their need for food and cater to any digestive issues that arise with the withdrawal of the old habit.

Since the individual will have a tough time regulating their hunger and stopping when they're full, it is best to seek professional help of a dietician or nutritionist to help them get started with foods they can eat and foods they need to stop binging on. Only when the repeated behavior of eating stops, can bulimia be treated.

Avoidant Restrictive Food Intake Disorder (ARFID)

It is an eating disorder characterized by a continuous failure to meet standard nutritional or energy levels which leads to one or more of the following issues.

- Significant weight loss
- Significant nutritional deficiency
- External feeding or dependence on oral nutrition

- An interference in psychological functioning

Causes

Like most eating disorders, there isn't just one culprit to place blame on. Although evolving studies have suggested that disordered eating breeds from multifaceted chemistry of sociocultural, genetic, and psychological factors.

Symptoms

Some of the most prominent signs and symptoms observed in someone living with AFRID includes:

- A limited list of eat-able foods
- Choosing to eat foods with similar characteristics such as colorless or crunchy
- Avoiding fruits, vegetables, and proteins
- Elimination of certain food and vowing to never eat them again
- Strict preferences on how their food is prepared
- Skipping entire food groups
- Food limitations which affect their social behaviors
- Demonstrating stress and anxiety when presented with something other than their preferred food
- Multiple nutrient deficiencies

- Poor weight gain

Where Intuitive Eating Comes In?

Changes are conceivable for people suffering from ARFID. Once intuitive eating is adopted as a means of treatment, it will help the patient with relying on internal cues in contrast to oral and external cues of hunger. Then it will also help in providing the patient with an abundance of nutrients in various forms such as raw fruits and vegetables, juices and dairy. This will also prevent significant weight loss which can lead to anorexia nervosa.

Binge Eating

We already understand what binge eating is all about as it has been discussed several times in the book earlier, however, since it is also an eating disorder, and fairly a common one these days with the whole Netflix and chill theme, it is crucial that we understand the long-term effects it can have on our digestion, metabolism, and overall health. Not only will the unusually large consumption of usually fun foods add to your weight, the amount of carbs and cholesterol in them also slows down heart rate, making one feel less active and lethargic throughout the day. Going on a binge is also linked to a bloated tummy and gassy stomach and an increased risk of gastric reflux, which is both painful and uncomfortable.

Of course, there will be some occasions when you can eat as much as you want and have as many meals you desire, but don't let it become a habit. A lot of people have trouble eating normally after the holidays when they have down some hearty eating. No wonder, so many people's New Year resolutions involve getting in shape and thus gyms and sports clubs get so many new clients in the first week of January. Besides, there is a limit to overeating, and the sooner you realize that it is getting out of control, the easier it will be for you to bounce back to your routine eating habits.

Causes

There are a number of contributing factors that make one want to binge eat and develop an eating disorder. These factors include:

Psychological Factors: Psychological factors such as depression, stress, and anxiety have been linked with binge eating. Those who happen to binge eat also have a difficult time coping with their emotions and feelings and thus eat as a way to deal with them. They also tend to suffer from low-self-esteem and dissatisfaction with the way they look.

Biological Factors: Binge eating may also be a result due to hormonal imbalances in your body. Have you changed your diet, your sleeping habits or your workout routine? All these can lead to hormonal imbalances and irregularities. It can also be genetic. If your family has this habit of consuming food whenever they can get their hands on it despite being full, then maybe you have developed it because of that too. Food addictions also run in some families where the mother or the father is obsessive about eating something particular and the child becomes an addict too.

Cultural and social factors: Traumatic experiences can also cause binge eating. For centuries, food has been a staple for comfort for humans. They eat when they are stressed so they distract themselves. Sexual abuse, history of torn family relationships or a bad breakup can all increase one's chances of turning to food for comfort. Social pressure also has a certain role to make one binge eat. The constant pressure from your family, friends, and peers to be a certain weight, shape, and height can be too much for someone and make them vulnerable and unable to stop eating.

Symptoms

Although being obese or overweight is linked to unhealthy food habits, it is a telltale sign that one eats past their fullness or binge eat. But can only obese people develop this disorder? Sadly, no. We all are at risk of developing it if we continue to eat despite being full and satiated. If you think you have been eating more than usual, then you might want to check out these symptoms below and hope that you don't have to nod to most or all of them. These include:

- Consuming large quantities of food over a short period of time, say every two or three hours
- Acknowledging that your hunger isn't controllable
- Eating when not hungry or past fullness
- Chomping down food rapidly without worrying about the consequences
- Going on diets every few weeks but with little success
- Feelings of disgust, guilt, shame, and depression about your eating habits
- Eating until uncomfortably full
- Eating alone or in secret

Where Intuitive Eating Comes In?

At its very core, binge eating stems from a biological reaction caused by deprivation around food. It involves responses like eating because you haven't had a certain thing in three weeks and when you finally get your hands on it, it is impossible to stop. So, we can understand it as a reaction to cravings, which intuitive eating can help overcome. Another response to binge eating is something like this: "Oh well, haven't I already screwed up enough? Look at my weight, another slice of cake can't hurt me more." This roots from the fact that one has lost hope in getting into a better and healthy shape with eating right. People who binge eat start believing that there is no going back to what they used to look like. This happens because they have already tried several diets that failed them, and they put on the lost weight sooner than they had anticipated.

Luckily, all these problems have been looked into by the originators of the intuitive eating plan. Dieticians, Tibole and Resch understand these responses very well and thus laid the 10 principles which cater to each of these problems individually. If the binge-eating craze is due to unmet cravings, then intuitive eating encourages to fulfill them, if it is due to lowself-esteem, then intuitive eating also suggests that the moment you start respecting your hunger and your body needs, you will see a significant difference in the way you feel, and when you finally start watching your weight going down on the scale, you will regain your self-esteem and confidence back.

Once restrictions over food have been dealt with, the rest of the problems will dissolve themselves.

Emotional Eating

Emotional eating is eating because you feel emotionally unstable. It usually is a reaction to dissatisfactory emotions like sadness, loneliness, depression or stress. Think of it as a means to suppress negative emotions and feel a little better about your situation. Although there isn't any harm to eat to fill a hole in your heart or to comfort yourself, doing so frequently can become a disorder and a bad one.

Causes

Emotions play a key role in how our body feels. When we feel low, so does our body. When we feel stressed, the body releases the stress hormone cortisol which only worsens the situation we are in. When we feel sad or depressed, it too has a negative impact on our body. So, to uplift one's mood and bring out some positively the brain triggers the craving for something comforting. Unfortunately, whenever we think about comfort, our first choice is food. Maybe it is because it is so readily available and requires little to no movement. And since the body is already feeling down, it doesn't mind either.

Symptoms

Although emotional eaters will let you know that they ate a whole cake or a bag of chips because they felt low or wanted to cry, below are some of the symptoms they also portray. These include:

- Bloated tummy
- Stomachache
- Weight gain
- Eating in secret
- Buying in bulk quantities
- Depression
- Worry
- Shame
- Anxiety
- Isolation and social withdrawal
- Poor skin
- Feel like giving up on everything
- Troubled sleep
- Fatigue and tiredness

Where Intuitive Eating Comes in?

If we go back to the seventh principle of intuitive eating, we understand how emotional eating can be controlled. The principle teaches us to respect our feelings and promotes eating only when one feels hungry. If only we abide by that one principle, emotional eating will be put to an end as you will realize that food isn't the answer to your problems and too much of it can lead to uncomfortable feelings such as gas, bloating, and even fatigue. The moment one realizes that these feelings arise because of eating inappropriately or in large quantities, there is a chance that they would like to give up and eat right.

Next, we also have a principle that teaches us to respect our bodies and honor our hunger. Abiding by them can also help those with emotional eating disorders.

Nighttime Eating Syndrome

It is ironic that despite being a completely different eating disorder from binge eating, all the midnight snackers are also binge eaters. The only difference between the two disorders is that in binge eating, one consumes large quantities of food at short intervals. The nighttime eating syndrome doesn't necessarily involve too much food consumption. It is concerned with the urge to eat in the middle of the night. There are many reasons why snacking after midnight isn't healthy. For starters, those who have the habit of getting up in the night and looking for food in the fridge have interrupted their sleep. Their brain doesn't get enough time to relax and recharge. They also report having difficulty in falling asleep after snacking. Our bodies are designed to begin the process of digestion and metabolism as soon as we take the first bite of our food. Secondly, we have always been advised to have the last meal of our day 2 to 3 hours before bedtime. If we think about it, we are depriving our bodies of both these and eating without being hungry or giving the body time to digest and metabolize. This also adds to our weight and one important reason why people who eat in the middle of the night are obese or overweight.

Causes

Researchers are still deliberating over what causes people to develop this disorder but there hasn't been much research-based evidence yet. Some contributing factors that play an imperative role include hormonal imbalances. When one suffers from a hormonal imbalance, their body doesn't fully function like it is supposed to be. Therefore, the cues of hunger and fullness are often messed up.

Another factor is the habit to have dinner late at night after staying up past midnight. This is quite common among college and high school students as they tend to spend nights studying and binge-eating on whatever is available. Since they are distracted, they often overeat and thus develop it as a habit.

On and off dieting is also responsible for the nighttime eating syndrome. Since dieters avoid eating much throughout the day, when night comes, their body feels deprived of nutrients and thus begin to crave for food. Sometimes the craving is so bad that it can wake you up in the middle of the night due to extreme hunger. The restriction to eat less in the daytime comes out as frustration and hunger at night. And when the snacking continues, it is very seldom that one loses weight and thus becomes even more disappointed and continue to binge eat.

Symptoms

Some of the most common symptoms observed in someone with the nighttime syndrome include:

- Evening hyperphagia
- Morning Anorexia
- Difficulty in falling asleep
- Difficulty in staying asleep
- Experience irritation, anxiety, depression, and agitation which worsens at night.

Where Intuitive Eating Comes In?

Since intuitive eating disregards the diet mentality and instead, promote eating what the body wants, sufferers of the nighttime eating syndrome can adopt the habit of eating everything when the body really wants it. It doesn't have to be tied with time. When body cues are given importance, one learns how to handle their hunger in a timely manner. So when you feel fed and satisfied throughout the day, you won't be craving to snack during the night. Another way intuitive eating may help is to reject timely constraints that one has to eat at a certain time only. Eating in reasonable quantities when hunger strikes can help with the elimination of the need to eat during the night.

How to Eat Intuitively with Dietary Restrictions?

What about people with food intolerances and allergies? Is intuitive eating not for them? Catering to intolerances and allergies are becoming one of the top priorities of many food giants and restaurants. Many even go as far as developing a special separate menu to cater to just those with intolerances and allergies, which is great! But does that mean those with intolerances can't practice eating intuitively? Certainly not!

Here's how someone with, say a lactose intolerance or peanut allergies can continue with the intuitive eating approach and lead a healthy lifestyle.

Recognize Your Limitations

The first step to any disease, be it mental or physical is to accept that you have it and then move onto working towards the other courses of prescribed treatments. The same is the case with people with food restrictions and allergies. The first step is to recognize that you have an intolerance or allergy you have to be cautious about, no matter how frustrating it gets. But don't let that define all your food choices and you certainly don't have to be scared around your food either. Of course, you will have to work with them, but don't let them define you. There is still a lot that you can eat and enjoy to the fullest.

Focus on What You Can Eat

If you have an intolerance or allergy, only certain foods must be restricted. Now, you have two options here. Either you can continue harping that you have an allergy or deal with it and focus on the things you can eat. There is a wide spectrum of food groups and subgroups that you can enjoy. Why worry about that one thing you can't have and lose focus from the things you can have? If you still wish to, you can mourn the elimination of specific foods, but only for some time. When you are done, take a pen and paper and list down all the foods you can eat. We bet you will need more than just a paper or notebook to all the wonderful things you are allowed to eat without worrying about worsening your condition or having an allergic reaction. Once you have a list, notice how many foods you never tried or eat less of.

Satisfy Your Cravings

We all give in to our cravings at times. But what if the food you are craving is restricted? How do you go satisfying that when practicing intuitive eating which urges its followers to eat whatever they feel like and give in to the body cravings? Picture this, the person sitting next to you is enjoying a bowl of homemade pasta and all you can think about is diving right into it. But you are also gluten-intolerant which means it's a big no for you. How will you stop yourself and resist the temptation?

Here's how. Look for some substitute that is equally satisfying. Remember, if intuitive eating is about giving in to your cravings, it is also about eating healthy and feeling good about what you are having. Therefore, look for some substitute that brings out similar feelings from within like that bowl of pasta. It could be some fruits, nuts, a whole-grain item or something similar that you are tempted and excited to eat whenever you get the chance. It may or may not have the same effect on you, but you surely feel much better and satisfied after you eat it.

Focus on How the Food Makes You Feel

An important aspect of the intuitive eating program is how the food makes you feel when you eat it. The goal should be sheer enjoyment, joy, and satisfaction. There are many foods that can make you feel like a million bucks and those are the ones you need to focus more on. Whenever a temptation to have them arises, you don't have to resist it because intuitive eating teaches us so. Focus on how food makes you feel. Does it uplift your mood like ice-cream does for a kid or does it make you feel bloated and sluggish like a large bag of chips consumed in one sitting does to you? The more you understand how your body reacts to different foods, the better you will be able to nourish it with the best.

For someone with an intolerance or allergy, it is very convenient to hide behind them, but you have to change your behavior as well. Indolence doesn't have to limit you or make you follow a strict diet. In fact, it should open you up to trying foods you never tried before and develop a perception about them. Who knows you end up finding a bunch of foods you never tried before but ended up liking them? Besides, it also prevents feeling food-deprived and leaves with a more inclusive diet.

Take Away

In this chapter, we looked at the many different eating orders, learned about what caused them, pondered over the various symptoms patients depict and later dealt with the most pressing question about intuitive eating — how can someone with dietary restrictions can eat intuitively.

Chapter 6: Becoming an Intuitive Eater

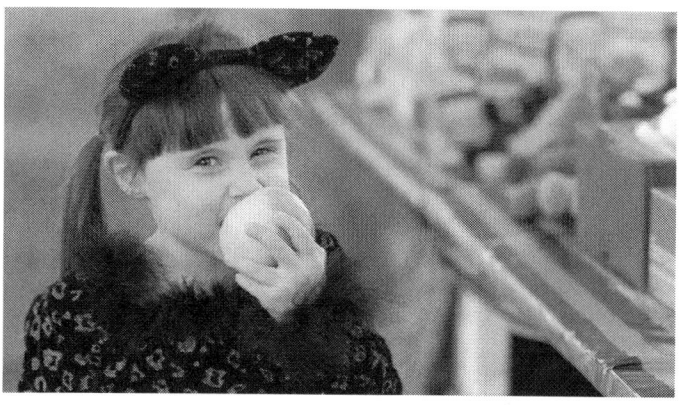

Eating intuitively is becoming a prominent and preferred way of eating today. Much of its hype is due to the fact that diets are failing people and they are finally realizing the harm it does to their body and mind. Be it the Atkins, vegan, keto or the paleo diet, their foundation is based on limitations and restrictions. It gets even worse when you jump from one diet to another simultaneously as it doesn't allow the body to get used to the new change when it had only begun to respond to the changes made prior.

The decision to diet involves more of our mental than our physical body. Who decides what our body needs and what it doesn't? The mind. Add to that societal pressure that keeps on projecting thinness as a beacon of beauty. But even then, it is up to us to decide what is best for us. Our thinking plays a key role.

When people decide to diet, they have a completely different mindset that promotes that thinking. However, since we are more interested in the mindset of an intuitive eater, let's compare both the mentalities and choose which one seems more sane, sustainable and suitable for you.

The Thought Process of an Intuitive Eater and Dieter

A Dieter's Mentality	Issue	An Intuitive Eater's Mentality
Do I Deserve it?	Food Choices and Eating	Do I want it? Am I hungry?
I am guilty when I eat fun foods.		Will it satisfy my craving for it?
I describe food as bad and good.		Do I like its taste?
Food is my enemy		I deserve to eat without feeling guilty.
My goal is to burn the calories.	Benefits of Exercise	My focus is on how exercise makes me feel.

	Viewing Progress	
I feel disappointed when I miss a day at the gym.		My focus isn't on how many days I work out but how energizing and stress-relieving it feels.
Do others think I look good or not?		I give inner body cues priority.
I have a strong willpower.		I have complete trust in myself and the food that I eat.
How many pounds have I lost?		My primary concern isn't losing weight but eating healthy.

You must have noticed the vast differences between the two mentalities. Firstly, where a dieter is more concerned about losing weight, an intuitive eater just wants to consume food that is healthy and nutritious. Secondly, there is no restriction of food and everything is allowed in an intuitive diet as long as it has good nutritional value and is satisfying. A dieter is rarely concerned about the satisfaction of the consumed food, meaning he or she is eating senselessly and thus depriving the body of not only a variety of nutrition but also taste and satisfaction. Thirdly, a dieter is always thinking about whether he or she should eat something, whereas an intuitive eater lets their body to decide if they want it or not.

If, as suggested by the above table, there is a difference between these two mentalities, then is there a possibility to jump from one to the other? Can a dieter become an intuitive eater if he begins to think like one?

Yes, but it is slightly difficult to change one's mentality completely when they are in adulthood. What were once just random conducts of action have turned into strong habits. Therefore, the only way to challenge them is with hard evidence.

Thus, it is best to start young and teach kids to be intuitive eaters during the developmental stages when they are forming opinions about things, learning, and forming habits.

Raising Intuitive Eaters

As discussed earlier, kids are intuitive eaters by birth. From the moment they are born, they have cried for food and had been fed. Then when they hit toddlerhood and began to differentiate between different foods, their taste, appearance, and smell, they demanded things of their choosing, which was, in fact, their body demanding them. With a few words to describe their needs, they were smart enough to tell their parents what they wanted. And when they felt full, they stopped. As fascinating as it was to watch them munch on their food, it is also important to note their likes and dislikes changed with time, even within hours. For example, has your child ever embarrassed you at a friend's or relative's house by eating something so delightfully that you told your friends and relatives that they hate it? You may have said something like, "Oh, my Timmy hates gummy bears. I tried so hard to get him to eat some but even the colors don't attract him." Moments later, Timmy is trying to fill his little mouth with as many gummy bears as he can fit making you come out as a liar.

However, you weren't a liar and you were right, he didn't like it, until today and that is because "he" felt like having them. Kids love to explore, and their exploration isn't limited to putting their fingers into places they shouldn't be. They are fascinated by their food as well. One day they cry the whole day for some boiled peas and wouldn't even touch one the next day. As parents we think, what the hell, and deliberately try to push them into eating them. What we are doing is taking away their intuitiveness. The ability to decide what their body needs with something that "we" want them to have. It is understandable that as their parents, you want the best for them, but what if we tell you that they are a better judge of it than you are?

Even we as kids were once intuitive eaters. We troubled our parents during feeding times because we weren't hungry, and they were determined to make us eat every last food on the plate. Somewhere in between that, we all grew up. Instead of listening to our bodies, we listened to those who seemed like experts at food and nutrition and changed the way we used to think and feel about our food. And that is when the problem actually began.

Food rules don't always begin at home. They can also form in places other than home such as our schools. Remember the time when the teacher wouldn't allow us to leave the table until we had finished our lunch? And there was a specific time allotted for the break which meant that if you felt extremely hunger before the lunch break, you were allowed to eat food and if you didn't feel hungry during the lunch break, you were still asked to finish your lunch? Sounds unfair, no? Add to that the rewards we were promised. "Honey, if you finish your food, daddy and I will take you out for ice cream. You like ice cream, right?" Bribery worked its magic and despite being full, we were forced to overeat. These are examples of how we have been interfering between our kids and their bodies. We have changed their eating behavior to meet a standard only to realize later, that it was a mistake. So, if it happened with you but you don't want your child to go through the same, below are some great ideas to raise your kid as an intuitive eater and promote behavior that allows them to listen to and put their body needs first.

How to Raise Your Kids to Become Intuitive Eaters?

Be a Good Teacher

Who, according to you is a good teacher? Someone who knows what he or she is doing or someone who is just reading from a book? Someone who believes and lives by the values they teach their kids every day or someone who is just concerned with the end result at the end of the course?

In order to teach your kids how to become an intuitive eater, you must become one first. You have to heal your relationship with food first so that you can know how they will feel and respond to the new changes. Besides, we all know that kids are great imitators. They do as they see others doing. And who are better role models than parents themselves?

Thus, if you want them to eat intuitively, you need to teach them by example. Your kid looks up to you in all aspects of life. So, if they see you restricting yourself from certain foods, they will think of them as distasteful too. Likewise, if you don't feel good about yourself, the way you look, and your food choices, then chances are they too will pick up on the negativity and think of themselves the same way.

When you are around your child, avoid labeling different foods as good or bad. If they want sweets, don't tell them that it will lead to a toothache. If they want a bag of chips, don't scare them by telling them that will cause their stomach to ache. You must remove all feelings of guilt and shame towards foods. Intuitive eating teaches us that there is no such thing as good or bad food, and we must tell them the same as well.

Aim for Balance but Allow Them Options

Allow them to have food with different textures, colors, and shapes. It is all about what sparks the most fascination for a kid. Since they love to explore new things, a variety of things to choose from will make mealtimes more enjoyable for them. Include a combination of fruits and vegetables or nuts and dairy. And don't get upset when they eat some of the things on their plate and leave others. What better insight would you have than knowing of their preference? If you are trying to make them an intuitive eater, you just need to add more of the things they ate the next time around, even if they weren't the most nutritious of foods. Intuitive eating doesn't restrict any foods and the different combinations will only make it easier for you to understand what your child likes and doesn't like.

Don't Stop Offering

Gaining a preference over their favorite foods is going to be a long process. Think of the foods as reality show contestants. They all have their own skills and talents, but it is only the judge that chooses the best out of them and says bye to the remaining one. Try offering your kids something new every day so that they can pick. The key is to never stop offering something new or intentionally placing on their plates, the foods that were rejected the last time. Although it is a nice tactic, it doesn't guarantee results. What if your kid eats it now because he or she is super hungry but doesn't even look at it the next time because they have other things on their plate too.

Another important thing for parents to know is to encourage the use of words like crunchy, sour, sweet, and soupy to describe food. The next time you ask them, and they tell you that they want crunchy, give them foods that fit that description. This will encourage them to eat when foods are grouped into different categories. To make things more interesting, try presenting it in playful ways such as assorted by color or arranged in different shapes or placed on the plate according to their sizes. Not only will it make their mealtime more interesting, but it will also be something that they can learn from.

Mind Your Language Around Food

How you speak about different foods is important as kids pick up things very fast. Labeling things as good or bad will only lead the kids into thinking about them in a judgmental way. Instead, try using words like fun foods or growing foods instead of junk food or healthy foods. Since your goal is to make them an intuitive eater, labeling something as bad will add a negative connotation to it.

Let Them Be the Judge

As parents, we all want to offer our kids the best that is out there. However, sometimes we feel like despite their favorite things being placed right in front of them, they seem disinterested. You keep trying to push them into eating and they do take a few bites, but it seems more forceful than enjoyable. Let your kids choose when they want to eat and what they want to eat. Trying to force the idea that they are somehow bound by a time constraint is wrong. Have you ever eaten a big meal for lunch and didn't feel like eating dinner? The reason you didn't eat at dinner time is because your intuition told you that you weren't hungry. The same thing happens with kids. They are born with the same intuition, so let them use it wisely.

Conversely, if a kid keeps on asking for something every few hours, then don't shush them and tell them they can't have it now because there is only an hour left for dinner. Kids are experts in their own bodies. Maybe the previous meal they ate was digested faster. Perhaps they had a busy and active day and thus their body needs some more energy to keep going. The point here is, don't question their motives for eating. If they say they are hungry, they probably are. The same applies to when they tell you that they have eaten enough. Don't try to force-feed them what's left on their plate or in their bowl.

Lastly, if they have a bad feeling towards certain vegetables, don't force them to eat them. This will set a negative connotation towards those vegetables and your child will always throw a tantrum when they are presented again. Of course, your intentions are to feed them with good nutrition but let that be for some other day or time.

The Holiday Survival Guide When Eating Intuitively

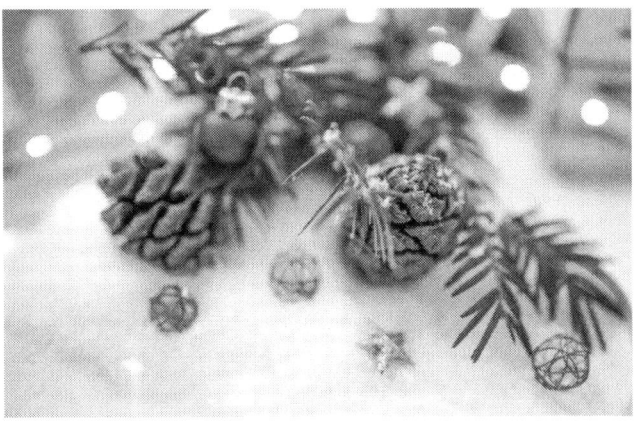

Holidays are that time of the year when we are bombarded with texts from friends and family, planning our holiday dinners, and checking our availability. However, you just starting intuitively. How are you going to handle the delicious starters, the devour-able entrees, and the sweetest of desserts? You already had a little too much around Halloween and swore that you wouldn't get into that eating frenzy ever again. What are you going to do to control your eating when literally everyone is insisting that you take some more?

Well, for starters, intuitive eating has never stopped you from eating the things you love. Of course, there are a few limitations like stopping when you are full but that doesn't mean you ditch the desserts variety completely. There are multiple ways to manage your cravings around food, even during the Holidays.

Most of us fall for the old dieting patterns thinking we will be eating too much around the holidays and gaining weight. True, there is this possibility and also that no matter how hard you try, you will still be tempted by everything that is presented in front of you. So are you going to worry about your weight or miss out on the delicacies until next year?

To help a diva like you in distress, we are presenting you with a number of ways you can keep eating intuitively without having to worry about gaining a few extra pounds here and there. Keep in mind that this time of the year is supposedly the most joyous one and your body deserves a treat too.

Visualize

Visualize how you are going to spend your time during the holidays. Think about what you will be wearing, who you will be talking to, how you will respond to food, how much you will eat, and how you will feel after eating it. The more detailed your visualization, the more prepared you will be to live that moment. Think of it as a rehearsal before an actual event. It only makes you more confident and in control.

What visualization will do here is to get your mind off of food and the worry associated with it. When you have a little plan of action about how you are going to approach food, how much you are going to eat, and how it will feel when you have it, it will make it less focusable. You will then be more concerned about meeting your family and friends and enjoy your time with them. You won't worry about whether you need to go for a run the very next day or not. Instead, you can act a little relaxed because you have it all under control.

We are most worried when we are faced with an uncertain situation — something we didn't plan for. However, thanks to visualization, the stress around food and whether you will be able to control will be minimized and prevent any emotional eating.

Create a Few Mantras

Next, you need to create a few mantras of your own to get you by the holiday season. Whether you like it or not, there will be someone discussing a new diet they found extremely helpful to shed weight or a new drink or supplement that makes you cut down on food, so you won't feel hungry all day. It is unavoidable and likely to make you impatient for two reasons. First, you are eating intuitively which means there is no restriction or limitation to what you can eat and second, you will be worried that your intuitive approach towards eating will be mocked and laughed at because it is not a diet, just normal eating. But remember, how you respond is up to you. You can either feel bad about your eating habits or completely dismiss their eating approach. So, every time you are faced with some backlash or forced into a conversation about food, chant to yourself something like, "I don't need to listen to this" or "It doesn't concern me, I should keep doing what I am doing." Doing so will serve as a reminder that you aren't wrong and don't have to listen to some gibberish all night just because you reject the diet mentality.

Secondly, you might also come across people who wouldn't stop gloating about how much miles they jog every day and that you should definitely try it sometime too. There is no forcing in intuitive eating. You aren't in a herd. You won't do what everyone else is doing. You will jog the day you feel like it, and more importantly, when your body feels like it. Again chant your mantras in your head and you will reassure yourself that you are doing well for yourself and your body.

Focus Your Energy and Time Elsewhere

Again, if you keep all your focus on what you are going to eat and how you are going to control and stop when you're full, then you will miss out on all that is happening. If the thoughts of food still haunt you, try distracting yourself by conversing with people. The more involved you are in the conversation, the less likely you are going to think about food. Thus, try engaging with people as it will help you drown out the voice in your brain worried about whether it will be chaos when the food is served or not.

Your goal should be to respond to food and not just react. You need to eat mindfully and not just try everything out of fear. And when the food is finally served, use the opposite strategy and avoid any conversations as it will only take your mind off of how much you have actually eaten, and you will miss your internal cues for when you are full.

Note That Feeling Little Too Full Is Acceptable

If, however, for some reason you do end up overeating, there is no need to start panicking. You haven't broken any rules. You just have eaten a little beyond your fullness. Intuitive eating is also about experiencing foods and if something feels so good that you have to request for seconds, don't regret it later. If it was worth it, then there is no point stressing about it. Don't start planning your next workout routine or promising yourself that you would skip all the following events until you have burned the extra calories. More importantly, don't give up on eating intuitively thinking you aren't worth it. It is okay to go over your eating intake. It's not like you will gain weight in a single sitting. Stressing will only mess up your mood and mental health.

Allow Yourself to Eat

Lastly, you have permission to eat. You need to verbally remind yourself of that, especially when you are trying to hold back onto something. Remember, you aren't following a diet anymore and have the liberty to eat whatever you feel like eating, even if that means stuffing yourself with stuffed chicken with oozing cheese. You have to allow yourself to enjoy food without judgment, otherwise, there is no point in eating it. Tell your body that it is allowed to eat whatever it craves, any time it wants, and until it feels full. Doing so will take the regret out of food and make your holidays less stressful and more enjoyable for you.

Take Away

In this chapter, we looked at the many different aspects of intuitive eating starting from the differences between the two mentalities — a dieter's and an intuitive eater. After stressing on the need for intuitive eating, we later delved into how parents can raise kids that are intuitive eaters and avoid the mistakes they usually make.

Lastly, as a bonus, we looked at how one can carry themselves during the holiday season which tends to be the most exhausting for anyone who has just started to eat intuitively. The practices include everything from distracting yourself from food to accepting that it is okay to eat without guilt and shame.

Chapter 7: Intuitive Eating and Weight Loss

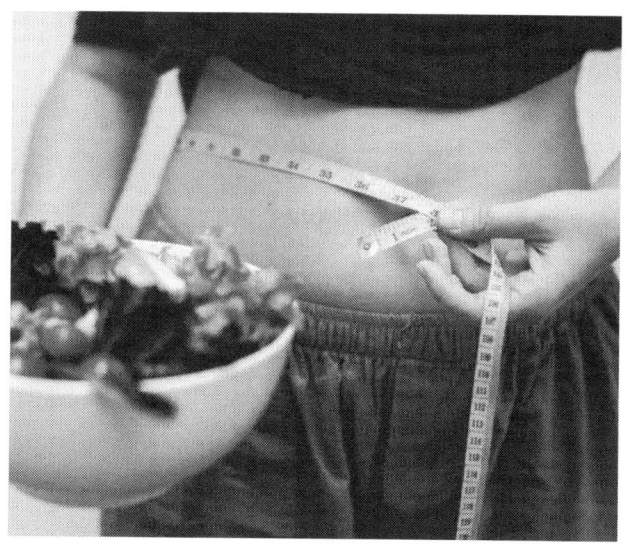

Unlike any diet, the core essence of intuitive eating isn't weight loss. It is more about addressing the different ways we eat. So, if someone has had a positive reduction in their weight with intuitive eating, good for them. But that doesn't mean everyone will feel the same or be greeted with the same outcome.

Although the possibility of intuitive eating leading to weight loss is still debated and there are different schools of thought. Since it is a fairly new way of eating, there is still room for more research and experiments to confirm this hypothesis. In this chapter, we are going to be discussing some of the most prominent and promising research studies and experiments that prove that intuitive eating does have promising results when it comes to one's weight maintenance, body image satisfaction, higher self-esteem, and better emotional functioning.

How Listening to Your Body Can Help You Lose Weight?

Traditional dieting programs have proven ineffective in promising sustainable results in the long run. It is quite common that lost weight is gained in less time once the dieting stops and the restrictions are uplifted. And that isn't even the worst part about them. They also happen to leave behind multiple psychological traumas such as anxiety regarding food, binge and emotional eating, and feelings of guilt and shame later. Such eating patterns are no good to anyone, especially someone who is trying to reestablish their relationship with food.

According to a study published in the *Journal of the Academy of Nutrition and Dietetics* titled *A*

Review of Interventions that Promote Eating by Internal Cues, researchers, Magnuson and Schafer, reviewed all the former studies around intuitive eating. All quasi-experimental controlled trials, randomized controlled trials, and cohort studies were reviewed. The goal of the research evaluation was to determine whether internal hunger and fullness cues, pleasure, satiety played any key role in weight management, weight loss or developing a healthier relationship with food or not.

The authors further reviewed all articles containing the terms intuitive eating, non-diet, mindful eating, attuned eating, and even health at every size intervention approach to eating.

After a thorough study of each and later selecting only the most relevant studies, the authors found 24 studies and articles that were later included in their final review. As per their findings, it was collectively concluded that patients who were previously obese or overweight and then looked at intuitive eating as a savior did report significant decreases in their weight.

According to a 2013 report published in the *Journal Appetite* by National Eating Disorder Association, approximately half a million young adults suffer from disordered eating and disrupted sleeping patterns which affected their skin, body functions, and energy levels. The most prominently observed disorders included compulsive eating, emotional eating, restrictive eating, obsession with certain foods, etc. Surprisingly, when a sample of 2,287 teenagers was studied, the researchers tried to study their eating habits. It was revealed that those who let their hunger cues determine their need for food intake were less likely to fall into the despair of eating disorders. They also reported better sleeping patterns and elevated energy levels compared to those who listened more to external cues than their own.

A research paper published in the *American Journal of Health Education* studied the meaning of food, the role of intuitive eating, and the relationship with the two versus diet composition. Intuitive eating proved to be a viable and sustainable approach to maintaining a healthy weight. The research survey included 343 university students who were asked their opinion regarding the intuitive eating scale and other diet-related scales. These were the conclusions drawn after an evaluation of their answers.

- Students that scored higher on the hunger and fullness (intuitive scale) reported lower BMI.

- Students who scored higher on the hunger and fullness scale also reported being less health-conscious when it comes to their relationship with food.
- Students who scored higher on the hunger and fullness scale also seemed to value the pleasure that comes from eating and food and reported higher levels of satisfaction.

To conclude, those individuals who gave their inner cues more value reported a healthier relationship with food and were less concerned about their weight management as compared to those who had been dieting. They also reported less anxiety around food and cared less about calories and more about how the food made them feel.

In another study published in the *Journal of American Dietetic Association*, researchers tried to figure out if intuitive eating helped one deal with size-related issues and led to the acceptance of the way they looked or not. The objective of the research was to determine how effective health at every size approach was and whether it helped people in improving their health or not.

Health at every size serves as an encouragement to eat intuitively and develop homeostasis regulation. A group of 78 females who were in the obese category were called upon to participate in a study. All of them were chronic dieters in their 30s and 40s. They were all asked to attend a six-month program including weekly intervention called the Diet Program vs. Health at Every Size Program. The clinical trial was followed by a six-month aftercare support group.

Throughout the study, the following measures were evaluated:

- Anthropometry
- Metabolic fitness
- Eating behavior
- Energy expenditure
- Attrition
- Psychology
- Participation and attendance in the study

It was noted that attrition was the highest in the diet group being 41%, whereas there was only 8% in the health at every size group. After the intervention, the diet group did show some swift improvements in multiple variables; however, it was only short-lived. In fact, they regained the weight they had lost and the improvements they had shown weren't sustained in the coming years.

On the contrary, the health at every size group not only maintained their weight in the next two years, but they also showed sustainability in the overall improved variables. So to conclude, it can be said more promising results were observed in those who had health at every size approach towards eating. The changes they made over time with intuitive eating were far more sustainable in the long run.

Another groundbreaking study consisting of different groups of teenagers proposed that intuitive eating can lower the risk of developing eating disorders like binge eating, midnight snacking, and emotional eating and also alleviate their symptoms. Compared with traditional means of dieting, which only makes one more worried about their calorie intake, this serves as a refreshing reminder that those battling eating disorders can switch to intuitive eating to prevent their onset and progression. Disordered eating has been reported to increase one's risk of developing multiple health conditions including blood pressure, stroke, obesity, and digestive problems. It also has a psychological impact and linked to increased anxiety and depression in many.

Although it is too early to say, intuitive eating does have many perks that no other eating approach offers. But of course, more research needs to go into finding how it actually works and how it can be adopted as the only approach to eating healthy.

Chapter 8: Intuitive Eating FAQs

As someone trying out intuitive eating for the first time, there must be many boggling questions on your mind regarding this non-diet mentality and whether this is the right approach for you or not, especially if you have been dieting religiously and just looking for an alternative approach this time around. Luckily, in this chapter, we are going to be answering some of the most pressing and obvious FAQs regarding intuitive eating for those in search of them.

So without further ado, let's get answering!

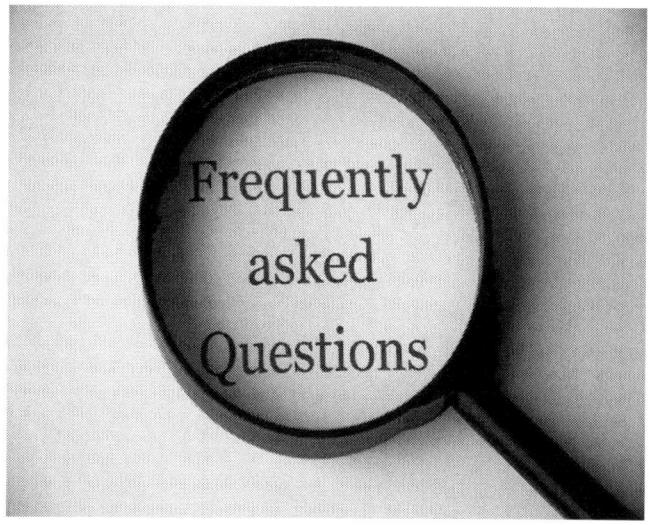

Is IE a Diet?

Sadly, no!

Instead, intuitive eating is a response to the diet mentality that strongly opposes the diet culture. There are no stringent rules and regulations that you must follow but there are 10 principles that teach you how to practice intuitive eating. The term was coined by two California-based dieticians Evelyn Tribole and Emily Resch, who after dealing with many diet-focused clients decided to publish their findings to help people get over the diet culture and focus more on building a sustainable relationship with food.

Where all diets tell you to abstain from a certain food group, there is no such limitation in eating intuitively. You also don't have to restrain yourself from any cravings you might have as intuitive eating allows its followers to consume whatever they like, in whatever quantity they like and whenever they like. This recognition of zero food rules is what makes it so unique from any other diet in the world and thus more doable. The majority of the work required to eat intuitively is to give up the former rules you abided by when you were dieting, which is easier said than done but possible.

Am I doing it right?

If you are treating intuitive eating as a diet, then there is a chance that you are doing it wrong. Here are some of the signs that you need to change your approach and start eating right.

- If you still feel like you have to hold yourself back from certain foods, then you are doing it wrong. Intuitive dieting is against restrictive eating behaviors.
- If you are still worried about the calories in everything and counting them mentally before every meal, then you are not eating intuitively. You need to stop focusing on the calories in everything and enjoy it. Also when you are too focused on counting the calories, there is a possibility that you won't be able to spot your hunger cues and overeat.
- If you are calculating the results by weighing yourself daily, then you aren't eating right. Intuitive eating is more about sustainable weight than weight loss. True, it does help some lose weight, but it isn't the actual goal. So, if you started eating intuitively thinking it will help you shed a few pounds and get you in shape, then you

began with the wrong idea and may be disappointed with the results.

Does it Work?

It comes down to your definition of the word "work." What was the goal you began with when you first started eating intuitively? Was it to build a healthy relationship with your food or was it to lose weight? One of the biggest dilemmas with intuitive eating is that people measure their success by the weight they lost rather than an improvement in their eating habits. They think that as long as some diet is allowing them to lose weight, it means it is working and vice versa.

Intuitive eating is more concerned about listening to your body's needs and leading a happy and mentally strong life free from guilt, shame or judgment of any kind. If this fits your criteria for what you mean by "working," then yes it works remarkably well.

What if I also want to lose weight? Is it ideal for me then?

If weight loss is your ultimate goal, then it may or may not help you.

As stated above, intuitive eating is more of a philosophy than a diet that encourages us to pay attention to our body's needs. It preaches to us to look for inner cues and schedule our meals. It promotes satisfaction that can only come from enjoying our meals to the fullest. It tells us to stop eating when we are full and never indulge in unnecessary overeating. It reminds us that it is okay to crave certain foods and that we mustn't deprive our bodies of them.

So, to say whether it will affect you or not and help you lose your desired weight is a very difficult and personalized question. Even the diets we follow demonstrate different results on different body types. Some people only lose water weight, while others are down by 10 pounds.

Since the goal of intuitive dieting is to break the chain of endless diets and take people out of their miseries of rollercoaster diets, it is very hard to tell if it will help them lose weight or not. There may also be times where you feel like you are gaining weight rather than losing it with intuitive eating. So, it is a matter of personal choice, to be honest. Ask yourself this, would you rather feel miserable and count every last calorie or would you like to stop worrying about that once and for all and stop skipping between different diets?

Your answer will determine if it is for you or not.

I fear that I will only eat junk if I start eating intuitively. How will I be able to stop?

Again, this is a very genuine concern that most people switching from a restrictive diet to intuitive eating is worried about it. True, this will be difficult but only because you are coming from a place where everything, but a few things were restricted. So, your first instinct would be to eat all the things that were once forbidden to your heart's content. There is also a chance that you won't stop eating even when you are full because you are so overwhelmed with how it is making you feel. This happens because your body has waited long enough to taste it and thus sends interrupted cues.

Secondly, after some time you will realize that you no longer feel the craving. Ask yourself would you like to have a donut on the seventh day as well as after the meal? If yes, would it still give you the same satisfaction it did on the first day you had it after so many weeks or months? Probably not! It is because you didn't hold yourself back from it and allowed your body to enjoy it as much as possible.

However, after some time the body begins to see it as monotonous and craves something else.

To answer your question if you will ever stop craving junk and eat healthily, then yes. You will although it will take some time to adjust to the new eating approach, so stay patient and don't lose hope.

Do I have to be driven?

Unlike any diet, there are no days, set timings or a list of things you can and can't eat. When you are bound by time and a number of days, you are more likely to stick around and feel motivated. It is the same as having a deadline to submit a report. When you take out that deadline you will possibly delay working on the report until the very last minute. Since there is an absence of a deadline or ultimate goal with intuitive eating, many may suffer from a lack of motivation, to begin with. Since it is eating like you normally would and everything you can, it can take some time to grow on you and make you want to continue with it. Until then, take your time and be patient. Even if you suffer from a lack of motivation, try not to give up and continue eating intuitively.

How will I know when I am hungry and when I am full? Is there some particular way to judge my fullness?

There is no secret formula to listening to your inner cues. You just need to practice and practice. We have already talked about the hunger and fullness scale. Try to place your level of hunger on it and see if you really are hungry or can still wait a few hours before eating something. The same applies to identify your fullness. Think of one on the scale as ravenous, four as neutral and 10 as full. The numbers may represent your hunger and fullness differently, but since you are just starting out, it is best to start with this. You can always adjust your numbers on the scale later based on your own preference. Also, each number is going to affect you differently. For instance, at level three, you may feel a growling tummy, but your friend might feel lightheaded. So everyone's scale is different. Moreover, it is best to avoid taking your hunger to a one as it may make you extremely hungry and you might end up overeating. Therefore, you must practice mindfulness at all times because the fullness cues are easy to miss. And Since the goal is to stop eating when you're full, you don't want to overeat and later regret it.

Lastly, let patience be your guide. It will take some time before you are able to exactly guess your hunger or fullness level. This is extremely hard for those who have been on restrictive diets as their hunger and fullness scale is messed up. But there is no need to be too harsh on yourself as it will only lead to losing your motivation and giving up on intuitive eating altogether.

How long before I become an intuitive eater?

This is a very subjective question as everyone's progress will be different. We all have our own timelines. You may have a hard time getting over something, while your friend may get over it in a few days or weeks. It all comes down to how well or poorly you react to change and how long you've been dieting for. The more damaged your relationship with food is, the longer it will take you to adapt to this approach. But even then, there is always a possibility of going back to your old practices, which means you will have to start from scratch altogether.

So, there can't be a definitive answer to this. However, if you stay true to yourself, allow your body to cue your hunger and fullness and abide by the 10 principles of intuitive eating, you will be astonished to see how quickly you are progressing towards a healthier lifestyle. Just keep in mind that since it isn't a diet, there isn't any expiration date or time.

If I am only eating junk what about my nutrition?

Believe it or not, there is a great likelihood that you will begin to eat more of what's nutritious and less of what is junk food. How will that happen? Picture this, you had a bowl full of mac and cheese only to realize that it made your tummy bloated and gassy. It isn't a nice feeling and if anything, the satisfaction you experienced while having it is minimized. Contrarily, if you had a bowl full of fruits or veggies, you are likely to feel lighter and more energized. Isn't that a better feeling than being bloated and gassy?

When you analyze the difference, you will want to eat healthier on your own so that you can avoid feeling uncomfortable later, even when the nutritious foods don't taste that good.

I have decided to eat intuitively but where do I begin?

First of all, congratulations to you for making the right decision to value your intuition to guide you from this point onwards. In order to begin, you must become familiar with the 10 principles of intuitive eating which form the basis of it. Secondly, you can seek help from a community of intuitive eaters and share your fears, struggles, and goals to feel like a part of a community. It is a fact that when people work in unison, they are likelier to achieve their goals. Besides, joining a community online or a support group can help you feel less stressed as you will always have someone to answer your questions and realize that you aren't the only one dealing with a particular issue.

There are also many books on intuitive eating which not only promotes the practice but also provides valuable insight on how to begin with the approach. Getting your hands on one of them can be extremely beneficial.

Take Away

In this chapter, we looked at the most commonly asked questions about intuitive eating. The answers are extremely helpful for someone still having a hard time deciding whether they should eat intuitively or take up another diet.

Well, look no further as this chapter answers all your queries in a detailed manner and help you get started with eating intuitively.

Chapter 9: The Benefits of IE

With over a hundred research studies swearing by its effectiveness, in this chapter, we are going to be talking about the benefits of intuitive eating — both the obvious and less obvious ones.

One Step Towards a Healthier You!

The biggest advantages of following the intuitive eating approach as opposed to any restrictive diet include:

- Decreased cholesterol
- Improved eating behaviors
- Decreased blood pressure
- Decreased body dissatisfaction
- Increased physical activity
- Increased self-esteem

These were some scientific researched benefits. Now coming to the less obvious benefits that most people fail to notice when introducing themselves to intuitive eating include:

You Are Able to Honor and Detect Hunger Cues

The best thing about intuitive eating is that it teaches us the art to detect our hunger cues so that we only eat when hunger strikes. This is a great way to honor the body. You are no longer restrained by time or eating mindlessly. You only eat when your body tells you to, even if it is right after you had a meal or late at night. Therefore, you must trust those cues and honor your body with what it craves.

You Are Able to Differentiate Between Foods

Since you aren't permitted to let your external cues decide what you should eat and when, you are no longer a captive to your own body and can feed it with whatever feels good. Since it isn't unlike any other diet, you have a free hand at exploring different food groups and eat things of your liking. With intuitive eating, there aren't any forbidden foods that also cut down your need to binge eat, you did in the past. When all your cravings are met in a timely manner, you no longer feel deprived or eat more than you should which helps with maintaining your weight.

As you explore further, you realize that there are no good or bad foods and that each food has some purpose to serve. This also means that you can enjoy whatever foods you previously didn't know about or restricted yourself from.

You Become Less Guilty About Your Food Choices

There are less guilty feelings surrounding your food. You are able to put the food police to a quiet and eat without being worried about the consequences or how much exercise you will have to do just so that you can burn the calories you've just eaten. There is little to no judgment on your part as well. Doing all this allows you to actually taste your food and feel the effects it has on you.

Food Feels Better to You

When the feelings of guilt, shame or judgment are put to rest, you are finally able to enjoy your food as you should. You begin to eat more mindfully and give all your senses a treat every time you have a meal.

You Become More Aware

As soon as you begin to enjoy your food, you also start noticing the effects of different foods and how they make you feel. Some foods may leave you feeling bloated, while others just uplift and energize your mood. Once you are able to differentiate between food choices like that, you are more likely to eat foods that make you feel happier and elated rather than those that cause bloating and fatigue. This enables you to have a better and healthier relationship with food as you also become aware of your satiety cues.

You Don't Crave Things Like You Used To

This is probably the biggest advantage of intuitive eating. You are able to control and manage your cravings. Since the process of reestablishing trust with your body has begun, you are better able to honor your hunger and fullness by giving your body the things it really wants to eat. This means that you eat what your body requires which makes the onset of cravings less frequent. How? You are no longer restricting yourself from anything.

You Become More Confident About Food Choices

Your self-confidence also takes a boost. When you have established a healthy relationship with your body, minimized the guilt and shame and presented yourself with the opportunity to eat whatever you feel like, you become more confident about yourself. You realize that food is no longer the only thing that defines you and even if it is, then you have it covered. Life is no longer apologetic, and you learn to live it to the fullest. You no longer feel like someone else should be the judge of how you look or should look.

You Become Flexible

For any dieter, it can be both annoying and worrying when they are pushed to show restraint when they are with their friends or peers and forced to just take a break from their diet for just one night. Call it a hardcore dieter's biggest nightmare. Luckily, if you are practicing intuitive eating, you don't have to go through such dilemmas, and you are more open to accepting unplanned dinners and hangouts without feeling any guilt about them later.

You Begin to Enjoy Exercise

Since you are following all the principles of intuitive eating, you are also honoring your body with the right amount of physical exercise to keep it healthy and flexible. When you aren't worried about the numbers on a scale and just exercising because you want to, it stops feeling like a chore and becomes more enjoyable. The moment you realize that you are doing it to please your own body and not anyone else, the workout becomes enjoyable and less stressful. This happens because you begin to view exercise as a means of self-care and not a fat-burning regime. Therefore, if it ever happens that you aren't able to go to the gym or feel like taking a rest day, you won't feel any guilt or shame.

You Are Able to Enjoy Trigger Foods

Wait, did we just say trigger foods? All dieters must be losing their minds and turning pages because now they are craving one. This isn't the case with intuitive eaters as they are not only able to keep them in the house, they can also enjoy them whenever they like. However, since they have excelled at keeping their cravings at bay, there is no hurry to binge eat it all in a single sitting. Sometimes they even forget they have them in the first place which is a prime example of managing cravings.

You Are Able to Stop When You Are Full

No longer do you have to finish everything on the plate once you sense that you have reached the state of fullness. There is no longer any shame in leaving leftovers on the plate as you don't have any obligation to finish it all.

You Are Less Judgmental and More Curious

You begin to approach different foods with more curiosity and less judgment. You don't always have a mental battle with yourself about whether you should have it or not. Instead, you become more thoughtful and reflective. You take full responsibility for your actions and realize that you no longer have to beat yourself up about it or regret it later.

You Become More Receptive

You start trying foods you never tried before. This also includes all those foods you had restricted yourself from eating formerly. You are also more open and receptive to various cuisines. Think of it as trying out a random dish on a restaurant menu instead of scrolling through the menu online and counting the calories in each dish or wearing revealing and fitted clothes because you don't care what everyone is going to think. If you've reached this point in your life, then this is when you have fully adopted intuitive eating.

You Are Less Critical of Yourself

You learn of self-compassion and understand how important it is to feel comfortable in your own skin. You no longer are worried about losing weight or looking good in a dress; your prime concerns become enjoying your time and feeling the freedom that comes with intuitive eating. You also start caring for yourself and treat yourself with things you previously were too afraid to even try. Alternatively, you also stop beating yourself up about the way you look or how others see you and just feel like "you."

You Turn to Coping Mechanisms Other Than Food

What once was the easiest option is no longer an option anymore. While eating intuitively, you realize how damaging it was to eat mindlessly, driven by emotions and cravings. They no longer remain a viable coping mechanism as you know that giving in to the temptation of food will only make you regret it later and cause health concerns. Therefore, when a craving does arise or you are down with emotions, you look for other ways to overcome them instead of relying solely on food.

You Feel More Elated

There is a significant improvement in your mood. Since you have successfully eliminated all the guilt and shame associated with food, you no longer are fearful about your cravings or eating things that were once restricted. You become more concerned about how you feel physically and mentally and in general feel happier and satisfied with your choices.

You Feel Satisfied

In general, your life stops revolving around food, which means you have more space in your head to think about the other things happening around you. When you find yourself becoming an active part of conversations, you get good at relationships with others. This only adds to your satisfaction with your life as you are able to focus your mind and energy elsewhere. There is little stress or worry about what others think of you or the way you look which boosts your self-confidence and promotes happiness.

You Become Mindful

Mindfulness and intuitive eating go hand in hand. As soon as you begin to eat intuitively, you also become a mindful eater. There are hundreds of benefits of each and when you are practicing both at a time, you can imagine how many advantages you are able to get. You become more aware of the present and focus on what you are eating right now instead of worrying about your next meal. This also leads to more self-awareness about your body and you become better at addressing your internal cues.

Take Away

This chapter looked at the various ways of how eating mindfully can help us from lowering our cholesterol and blood pressure levels to promoting eating mindfully. It helps us improve our perception on how we look and helps us enjoy exercising. It also reminds us to cope with our emotions and feelings with things other than food to ensure us that trigger foods will no longer trigger us... All of this and much more have been discussed in this chapter to help you learn of the multitude of benefits IE offers.

Chapter 10: Is it For Me?

This is one of the most pressing questions everyone planning to make the big switch ask themselves every day. Although we have covered most of it in the FAQ section, if you still have a few doubts, here is our final answer to this.

Who Benefits the Most from Intuitive Eating?

If you are looking for a one-word answer then here it is — EVERYONE!*

*Of course, there are a few exceptions such as those who are diabetic or suffer from some other severe health issues like Crohn's disease. But then again, no other diet is good for them either as they can't simply eat whatever their gut tells them to. Other than that, some of the groups of people that can benefit the most with intuitive dieting include:

Dieters: Those who have or still choose to the diet can reap great benefits with intuitive eating. Since they mostly have to practice restriction with certain foods, they can get rid of them once and for all with intuitive eating.

Kids: Being naturally intuitive, kids growing up as intuitive eaters can be more in control with their eating behaviors and less likely to develop an eating disorder if they have been taught to eat intuitively from an early age.

Teenagers: Teenagers or college-goers are the biggest age group battling with eating disorders. The disorders arise due to several inappropriate eating habits such as binge eating, snacking up too much on fun foods, and interrupted sleeping patterns. Intuitive eating principles can help them build a better and more promising eating behavior as they grow older and step into the professional world, which, let's face it, is only going to be harder and more draining. Therefore, the possibility of neglecting food or adopting good food habits is rare.

Workaholics: Workaholics have a severed relationship with food. Their eating is usually clocked and consists of basically whatever they can get their hands on. There is no structure to their diets which can lead to multiple health conditions later in life. How can they benefit from eating intuitively? By listening to their inner cues and taking out the time to care for their body and mind by giving it some nutrition and rest.

Obese or Overweight: One of the biggest challenges to losing weight is abstaining from former habits. Since people who are obese have no rules to eating, this is the first thing they need to work on when they are trying to get in shape. How can intuitive eating help in doing so? Well, if you are looking for an answer now, you really have missed all the advice we served you within this book. Go back to the 10 principles and tell us that they aren't enough to motivate you to reassess your eating habits? As soon as you start eating intuitively, you will notice a change in your urge for foods and with time, you will realize that food isn't the only thing on your mind anymore. When that gets settled in, you will move forward with honoring your body and only indulge in foods that are gentle nutrition. And as soon as you start honoring your body, listening to the hunger cues and stopping when full will become easier.

Binge or Emotional Eaters: Lastly, binge or emotional eaters can benefit from intuitive eating as well. Since their primary way of responding to any situation, be it good or bad, is with food, limiting the amount they eat in short intervals of time or eating too much at a time can help them get back to having a healthy relationship with food and also help them get back in shape.

Intuitive eating is for everyone looking to build a healthy relationship with food. There are no exceptions whatsoever and everyone can reap the remarkable advantages it has to offer.

Conclusion

At first, the idea of using your intuition to help you figure out an eating approach best for you may seem scary and downright ridiculous. But you mustn't forget that we all were once intuitive eaters. It is all about going back to your roots and starting afresh, how nature wanted it to be like originally. As kids, we let our intuition and curiosity guide us and as it turns out, we did grow up to be good and healthy, then why fear to listen to it again? We ate when we were hungry, rejected eating more when full, enjoyed eating a few things and rejected the ones we didn't. Simple no?

It wasn't until we were indoctrinated and introduced to the diet culture popularized by a few big brands who one day decided to take control of our eating habits. Add to that the obsession with thinness and how it affected the lives of millions across the globe trying to eat in a restrictive way so that they can look a certain way.

Thankfully, with the advent of intuitive eating, we again have a chance to turn back time and eat like we were supposed to. So are you going to take that chance or not?

We hope that this book offers all the insights you had been craving for related to intuitive eating. It has the potential to make your life fulfilling, happier and more satisfactory. It has everything — a guide to starting out, the 10 principles to lead you, answers to all your mind-boggling questions and myths that needed to be debunked and how you can implement the approach to intuitive eating into your life.

Finally, if you enjoyed this book, then I'd like to ask you if you would you be kind enough to leave a review for this book on Amazon? It would be greatly appreciated!

Free Bonus

Thank you for reading this book.

I hope you find it insightful, inspiring, and practical and I hope it helps you to achieve what you really desire

To accelerate your journey **from today Go to link** http://bit.ly/IEbonus **to get a**

INTUITIVE EATING CHEAT SHEET

1 page printable PDF with
- **5 Steps To Get Started**
- **10 Principles to Live a Fulfilling and Diet-Free Life**

This will help you time your next meal and also allow you to keep track of your fullness!

Download the Audio Version of This Book FREE

If you love listening to audio books on-the-go, I have great news for you. You can download the audio book version of this book for **FREE** just by signing up for a **FREE** 30-day audible trial! See below for more details!

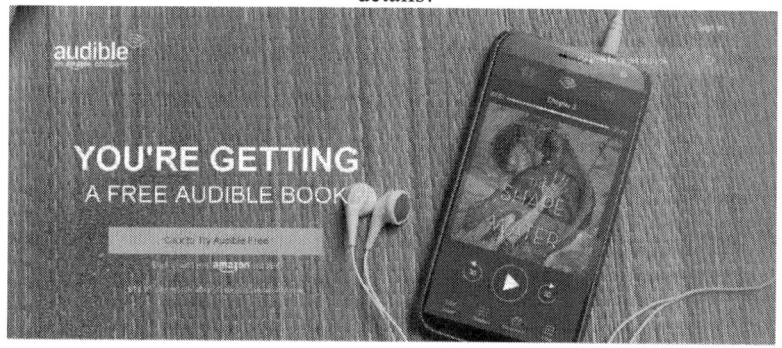

Audible trial benefits

As an audible customer, you'll receive the below benefits with your 30-day free trial:

- Free audible copy of this book + 2 Audible Originals
- After trial get 1 audiobook and 2 Audible Originals each month
- Choose from over 400,000 titles
- Listen anywhere with the audible app across multiple devices
- Make easy, no hassle exchanges of any audiobook you don't love
- Keep your audiobooks forever, even if you cancel membership
- Cancel anytime, no questions asked
- And much more

Go the links below to get started

For Audible US: https://adbl.co/38pBmAr

For Audible UK: https://adbl.co/2RAtg1i

References

10 Principles of Intuitive Eating. (n.d.). Retrieved from https://www.intuitiveeating.org/10-principles-of-intuitive-eating/

Abbate, E. (2019). 4 Reasons Diets Don't Work (And Never Will). Retrieved from https://www.shape.com/weight-loss/tips-plans/why-you-should-stop-restrictive-dieting

Bodak, C. (2017). 6 different types of eaters: Which one are you? Retrieved from https://www.fox19.com/story/34630196/6-different-types-of-eaters-which-one-are-you/

Graue, L. (2019). An exploration of differences between intuitive eating and mindful eating. Retrieved from https://www.fiercelyembodied.com/blog/an-exploration-of-differences-between-intuitive-eating-and-mindful-eating

Grabinsky, C., Matthews, D., Arnold, C., Marvel, P., Jure, J., & Cantwell, E. (2015). THE BROWNIE EXPERIMENT.

Harbstreet, C. (2019). What to Do About the Holidays When You're Working on Intuitive Eating. Retrieved from http://www.streetsmartnutrition.com/intuitive-eating-for-holidays/

Lauren Fowler. (2015). Intuitive Eating 101: How to Get Started. Retrieved from https://www.laurenfowler.co/blog/intuitive-eating-101

Malacoff, J., & Malacoff, J. (n.d.). Why Intuitive Eating Is Actually Really Difficult. Retrieved from https://www.shape.com/healthy-eating/diet-tips/intuitive-eating-problems-tips

Miller, K. (n.d.). The Real Reason You Don't Need A Diet. Retrieved from https://www.refinery29.com/en-us/diet-problems

Morrot, G., Brochet, F., & Dubourdieu, D. (2001). The Color of Odors. *Brain and Language*, 2001.2493.

Movara Fitness Resort. (2015). 7 Types of Eaters - What Type Are You? Retrieved from https://movara.com/7-types-of-eaters-what-type-are-you/

Nourishing. (n.d.). Retrieved from
https://www.lifespan.org/lifespan-living/five-myths-intuitive-eating

Peirano, J. (2017). The 6 Different Types of Eaters: Which One Are You? Retrieved from https://www.cheatsheet.com/health-fitness/different-types-of-eaters-which-one-are-you.html/

Please Quit Your Diet, Now. (n.d.). Retrieved from https://www.psychologytoday.com/us/blog/raising-happiness/201203/please-quit-your-diet-now

Psychology of Eating. (n.d.). Retrieved from https://psychologyofeating.com/the-science-and-psychology-of-intuitive-eating/

Psychology of Eating. (n.d.). Retrieved from https://psychologyofeating.com/intuitive-eating/

Rumsey, A. (2019). 24 Intuitive Eating Benefits: Alissa Rumsey Nutrition. Retrieved from https://alissarumsey.com/intuitive-eating/intuitive-eating-benefits/

Spanjers, B. (2018). The Biggest Misunderstandings about Intuitive Eating. Retrieved from https://barbaraspanjers.com/the-biggest-misunderstandings-about-intuitive-eating/

The 10 Principles of Intuitive Eating. (n.d.). Retrieved from http://eatuitive.com/blog/the-10-principles-of-intuitive-eating/

The Five Intuitive Eating Mistakes You're Making. (2019). Retrieved from https://www.ionlycameforthecake.com/five-intuitive-eating-mistakes-youre-making/

Wansink, C. (2005). The office candy dish: proximity's influence on estimated and actual consumption. *International Journal of Obesity*, 871-5.

Printed in Great Britain
by Amazon